bLaCK hAir

Art, Style, and Culture

Edited by
IMA EBONG

Foreword by
A'LELIA BUNDLES

UNIVERSE

First published in the United States
of America in 2001 by
UNIVERSE PUBLISHING
A Division of
Rizzoli International Publications, Inc.
300 Park Avenue South
New York, NY 10010

© 2001 Ima Ebong
Design by Melanie Doherty Design,
San Francisco
Jacket photograph by Matthew Jordan
Smith

2001 2002 2003 2004 2005 2006 /
10 9 8 7 6 5 4 3 2 1

Printed in Hong Kong

Library of Congress Catalog Card
Number: 2001089977

DEDICATION

This book is dedicated to my Mother for her profound insight, inspiration
and unwavering support in articulating a vision for a better world, and to my
father for the priceless gift of Africa.

*Black Hair: Art, Style and Culture is the culmination of a six-year journey. This book
could not have gotten off the ground without the following people, helping to inch the project along every step of the way, for which I am immensely grateful.*

SPECIAL THANKS TO

Most especially to my sisters Inyang and Enoh for six years of unwavering
support and encouragement. To my Publisher, Charles Miers for his broad
vision and perceptiveness, and for understanding the concept from the very
start. To Gena Pearson my editor for her fine editing, her support, and steer-
ing the project to a successful conclusion. To managing editor Bonnie Eldon
for keeping this project in mind and on track. To Ismael Cabigao for pushing
me to present my proposal from my first day at Rizzoli, and to AP for saying
"yes." I am also grateful to Marta Hallett for generous support and to Sonya
Beard for putting in many late nights to ensure a perfect text. I especially want
to thank everyone at Melanie Doherty Design for the sensitivity, imagination
and high talent applied to this project—thank you Melanie Doherty, Tina
Besa, and Trudi Michael. Illustrated books rise or fall on the quality of the
images and I want to thank the photographers, artists, and models that generously agreed to contribute to making this book happen. I am grateful to
Margaret Hitchcock of Ebony 2000 Salon for her nurturing hands and her
generous help on the fine points of styling hair. Thank you Alva Rogers for
graciously permitting me to use your photograph on the front cover. In partic-
ular Natasha O'Connor at Magnum Photos Inc, for her tireless efforts and to
A'Lelia Bundles for providing important images from the Walker/Bundles
Family Collection. I am grateful to Terri Gardner, President and CEO of Soft
Sheen Products, Inc. for permission to use Soft Sheen Posters, and also to
Gladyse Taylor at Soft Sheen for locating the artwork. Curator Mary Year-
wood and James Huffman of the Prints and Photographic division at the
Schomburg Center for Research in Black Culture for their professionalism and
kind assistance, and Tammy Lawson of the Art and Artifacts division at the
Schomburg for her help in securing images at the last moment. Thanks to
Eileen Perrier whose brilliant exhibition of photographs on the London Black
Hair and Beauty show I found out about at the last minute—I am particularly
grateful to her for sending me a choice selection of work from her exhibition
for this book. I wish to thank Jeanne Moutoussamy-Ashe for generously
allowing me to include the photographs of Winifred Hall Allen. Thank you
Annu Prestonia of Khamit Kinks Salons in New York and Atlanta, and to
Daryle Bennett of Zoli Illusions for their interviews, and giving generously of
their time. Thanks to Maude Wahlman and Deborah Grayson for help with
research and to Adrienne Ingrum for her advice, enthusiasm and support.
Finally, I would like to thank all the writers, poets and artists who generously
allowed me to use their work, and from whom I received much encouragement. A list of picture credits to all those who have contributed appears on
page 143–144.

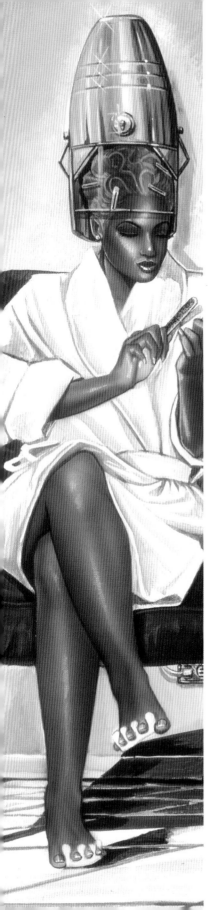

FOREWORD

From the once ubiquitous Royal Crown Hair Dressing tin—with its mildly odiferous scent and red, green and silver logo—to the coral-adorned ceremonial coifs of the royal women of Benin, Ima Ebong's enticing harvest of images pulsates from the pages of *Black Hair: Art, Style, and Culture.* Each photograph, painting and poem serves up another delectable morsel in this visual and literary feast of black women and our kinky, cottony, coily, wooly, wavy, wiry, croquinoled, cornrowed, straight, and straightened hair. Juxtaposing nineteenth Century African etchings of spiraled braids and bushy tendrils with the sky-soaring, ancestor-inspired hairstyles that currently crown the heads of black women from Los Angeles to London, Ebong confirms that the old eventually becomes the new. From the swirling strokes of artist Paul Goodnight's "Links and Lineage"—in which a mother, daughter, and grandmother bond through hair grooming—to the high fashion photography of a series of 1950s Madam C. J. Walker Manufacturing Company advertisements, she reminds us that our hair is art.

Through her eyes, our hair is also poetry, as in the words of Gwendolyn Brooks who captures both the sassiness of a 1940s upsweep "with humpteen baby curls" and the prideful strength of "rich rough right time" 1960s hair that shuns the curling iron. In these pages our hair becomes theater, too, breathed to life in George C. Wolfe's now-classic skit, "The Hairpiece," whose willful and warring wigs—natural-haired Janine and chemically coifed Lawanda—vie to be worn as their owner contemplates a break-up with a troublesome beau.

Having assembled the historical and cultural touchstones of our hair consciousness, Ebong moves a step farther, exposing the emotions that render one person's apolitical fashion choice yet another person's liberating political statement. "What's up with your perm, your locks, your blond extensions?" is likely these days to be answered with "Ain't nobody's business but my own what I do with my weave, my Goddess braids, my bottle of peroxide." From Patti LaBelle's towering hair sculptures to former Senator Carole Moseley Braun's regal braids to Mary J. Blige's golden tresses, we and our sisters improvise an aesthetic all our own.

With affection, honesty, and humor, Ebong—and the writers and artists whose offerings fill this anthology—celebrate our journey to love our locks—and ourselves—from Africa to the Americas. . . and back.

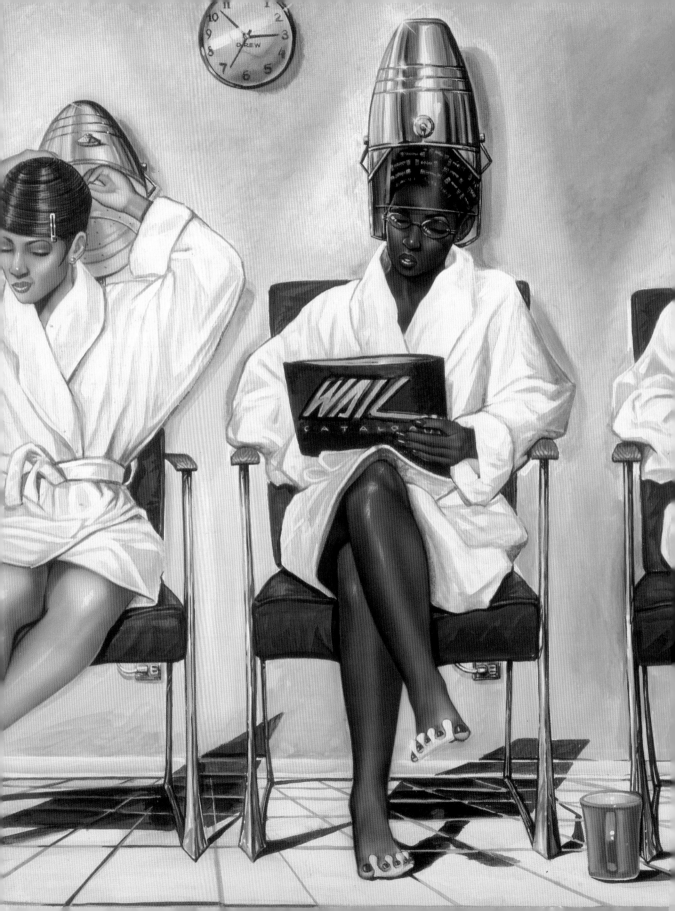

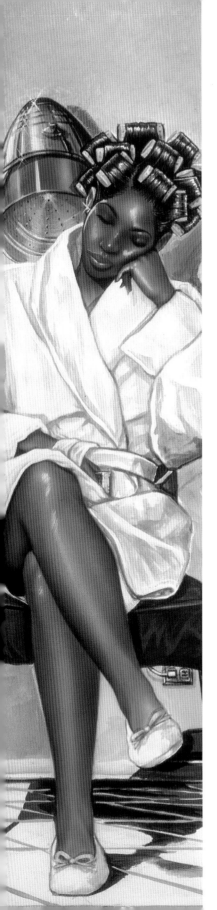

My visit to the hairdresser was a complete disaster, the kind that you may be familiar with. You slink out of your chair, pay your tip, and hope and pray that no one you know sees you on the way home. At such times, my usual strategy is to defy reality after the initial shock of seeing my new style. This is usually accomplished by avoiding the wall of salon mirrors, walking, eyes staring straight ahead through a gauntlet of equally horrified glances, returning only briefly to the scene of the crime to tip the offending stylist, then make a quick exit. On one occasion, in what was for me a small, yet important, act of rebellion, I refused to give the hairdresser a tip, the stylist not only lacked a sense of proportion (imagine Medusa meets the leaning tower of Pisa), but the final straw was her complaint that my hair was "not cooperating." How uncooperative could this multi-storied eighth wonder I was wearing be I wondered? It was the sort of hairstyle that not even hairdresser X, as we shall call her, would be caught with, but somehow it was her tour de force specially created for me. Needless to say stylist "X" became yet another addition to my blacklist.

Hair stories such as this and many others recounted here as excerpts of poetry and prose have been a staple of conversations among black women for generations. A visit to the salon is one of those moments of collective consciousness that could probably be appreciated by all women regardless of race, save for small details, like the endless waiting, plastic tubs of bleach bright white chemical hair straightener, or the familiar clang of hot curling irons snapping open and shut.

Black Hair: Art, Style, Culture is as much about the cultural ties that bind African women throughout the Diaspora as it is a recognition of differences that hopefully allow us to see ourselves in richer, more complex ways.

The open expressive Afro hairstyle for example, an icon of black pride and '60s activism in America in a wilder version becomes a symbol of mourning and an expression of grief for the Shawan women of Ethiopia. The elaborately coiffed towering hairdos so much a familiar sight at African-American hair shows and contests are juxtaposed with women of the Royal Court of Benin, with equally striking coral-studded hairstyles strictly designed according to rank and importance of each woman.

The advertisements, collected quotes, and other writings remind us of how we see ourselves, our frustrations, humor, and struggles to maintain this part of our being. Hair is an obsession, a statement, an object of gazing eyes and wagging tongues. Artists and poets, writers and dramatists have worked on this subject. The words and images presented in this book are a collage of past and present moments revealing an enduring fascination with hair.

Crown or glory, pride or problem, halo or hardship.

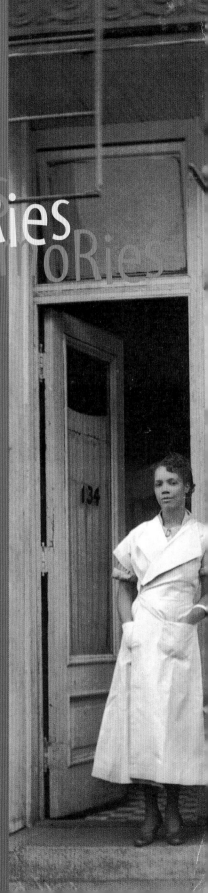

MemoRies

MemoRies MemoRies MemoRies MemoRies

"I asked my mother why,
since colored people were the only
people on the planet with hair like that,
why would they want to straighten it?"

Hilton Als, Hairstylist

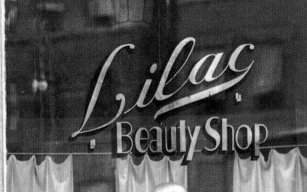

THE SHOP

Two spindly legs swimming in gray corduroy trousers made loose by frequent wear, the seat of the trousers made especially smooth from sliding in and out of the big, blue plastic chair with its square steel footrest. This was the chair her customers always sat in as she styled their hair, facing the mirror, facing themselves. At the end of those two legs—my seven- or eight-year-old own—my feet encased in down-at-heel black oxfords with round toes; they do not reach the footrest. When I tap the sides of my shoes together, hair falls from the soles, as if from a prehistoric monster's appendages, appendages given to shedding hair dyed red or gold or pressed by a hot comb.

The hair that falls does so as a result of my mother's handiwork in the beauty salon where she worked for a number of years. This was during the mid-to-late '60s. She referred to the salon in the East New York section of Brooklyn as The Shop. It was a storefront and dark; its interior was suffused with bright and brittle artificial light. It was also filled with women vainly trying—although they were often discouraged by the complicated effect, their appearance had on the world—to look like neater versions of their colored female selves, which a number of their employers and lovers considered something dirty.

In **The Shop**, there were a number of blue chairs and two black enameled sinks for washing color in or out. There were also bottles of blue liquid in which the combs floated like black plastic sea creatures with enormous grins and trays with silver hair clips (for bangs) and dull bobby pins (for curls) and brown hair nets that pressed down on coiffures, making squares.

The customers who frequented **The Shop** all seemed to want to talk at once. My mother and the two or three other beauticians who worked there (their employer did not do hair but kept her large round eyes—the exact shape and color of black ringlets pressed flat—on the books) would not respond much to their clients' talk, since they knew they were not meant to, not really. What their clients came for: as much to have their hair done as for the safety that greeted them upon entering that small room filled with women alone together, happily moored in their hairy harbor.

I do not remember how my mother felt about working in **The Shop**. But sometimes, in those moments when I am not at all resistant to memory's ability to sentimentalize nearly everything, I recall several of my mother's repeated actions as she worked in **The Shop**, my memory's favorite store: poking a finger into the jar of Bergamot; smearing a dab of the blue grease on the surface of her left hand; smearing the Bergamot between the parts she had combed in one or another woman's hair; click-clicking her single-barreled hot comb against its stiff metal base; colored crinkly hair being smoothed down by the hot metal in my mother's right hand; my mother waving the smell of burning hair and alchemy over to one side with her left hand, into thin air.

I would go to **The Shop** every day after school and wait a few hours for my mother to take me home. I did not like school at all at that time and considered it a place of enforced socialization. I already knew that my real life was going to be spent alone, not in isolation but as an observer. At **The Shop**, I could observe the emotional and intellectual exchanges of women coming and going, ostensibly to have their hair done but really to have a fleeting moment of safety in being themselves.

To be allowed to watch this felt like love to me.

After school on Friday, when my mother worked late, she would order takeout fried fish and chips for dinner — a special treat she bought for us with her tips, the coins and crumpled dollar bills that smelled like hair tonic. The crispy (on the outside) white fish was as crispy as the black or gold or red curls and bangs my mother made bounce on the heads of those colored women she knew wanted, above all, to be something other than themselves.

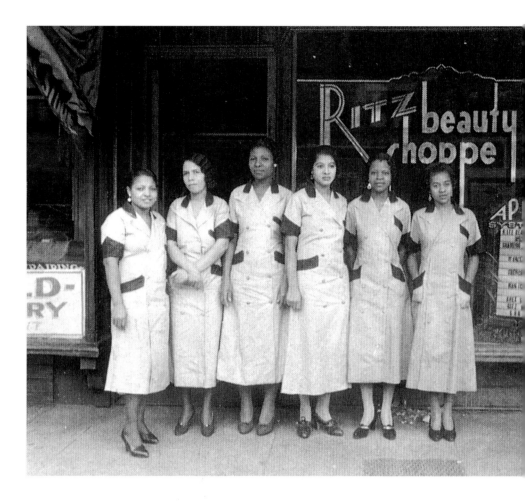

The two smells—the fish, the hair—mixed together in my mouth. My tongue, feeling satiated by all that good food and beauty, could not tell a lie.

I asked my mother why, since colored people were the only people on the planet with hair like that, why would they want to straighten it? My mother did not comment on this observation made by her most constant, nonpaying client; she only glared at me while tucking deeper into her fish or chips, not yet knowing that years after she had satisfied her appetite, and years before she died, **The Shop** would close down forever.

Hilton Als

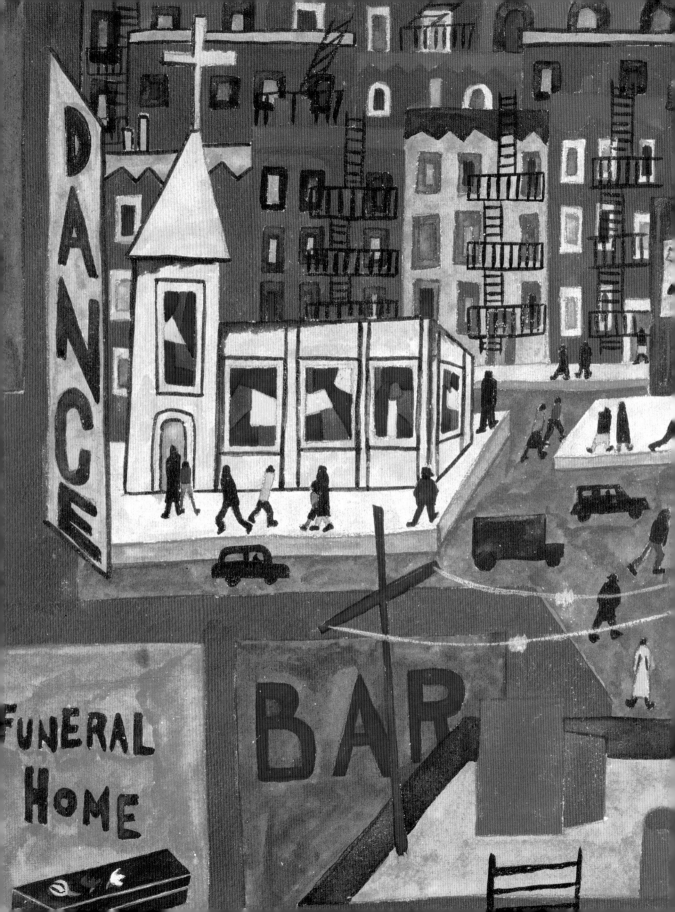

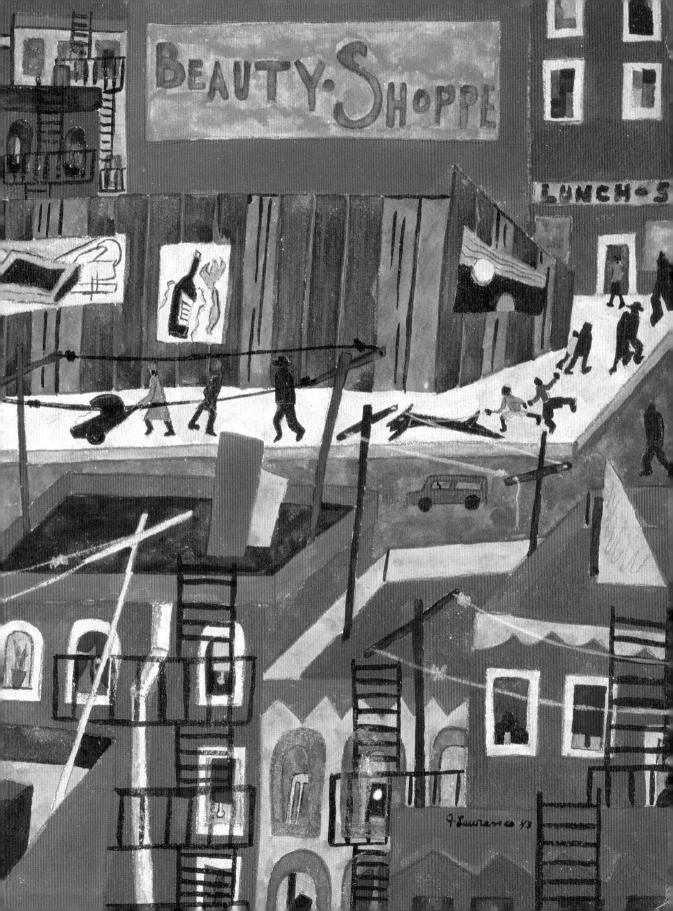

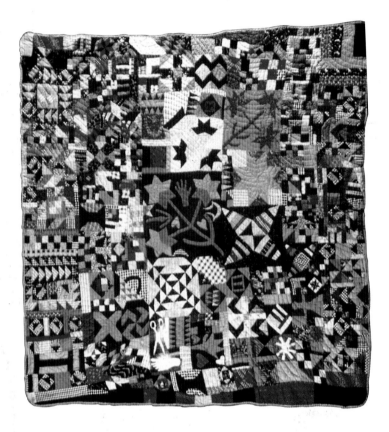

One of the scenes that did not, unfortunately, make it into the film [*Daughters of The Dust*] because of time—and there are so many of them—is a flashback to a period of slavery when Nana Peazant's mother cuts off a lock of hair and puts it inside of a small baby quilt for the baby Nana, who has been taken away from her and sold into slavery. The mother would send the quilt on to that plantation and when the child was old enough she'd be able to look in her own baby blanket and find a lock of her mother's hair. And sometimes that was the only thing that we had to share with our children or with our husbands and wives. They would send hair by messenger from plantation to plantation. And you know, during my research, I was brought to tears many times. I mean, if all you ever saw of your mother was a lock of her hair, that's all you had, and that's what you had to hang on to for the rest of your life.

Julie Dash

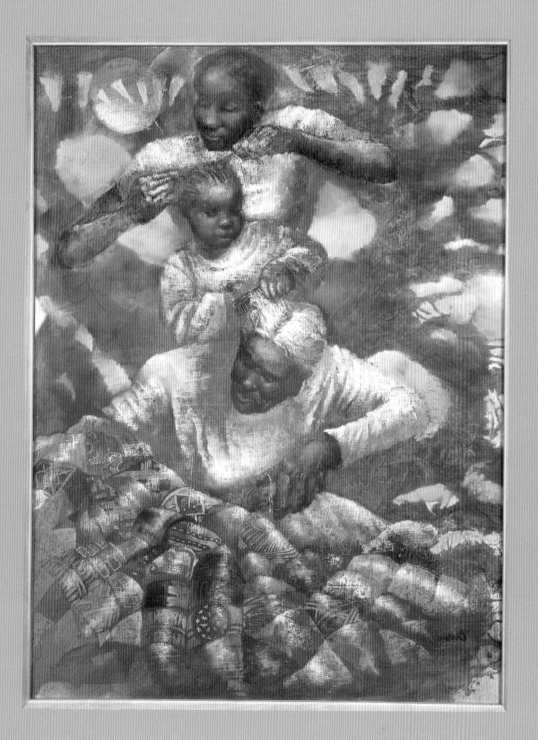

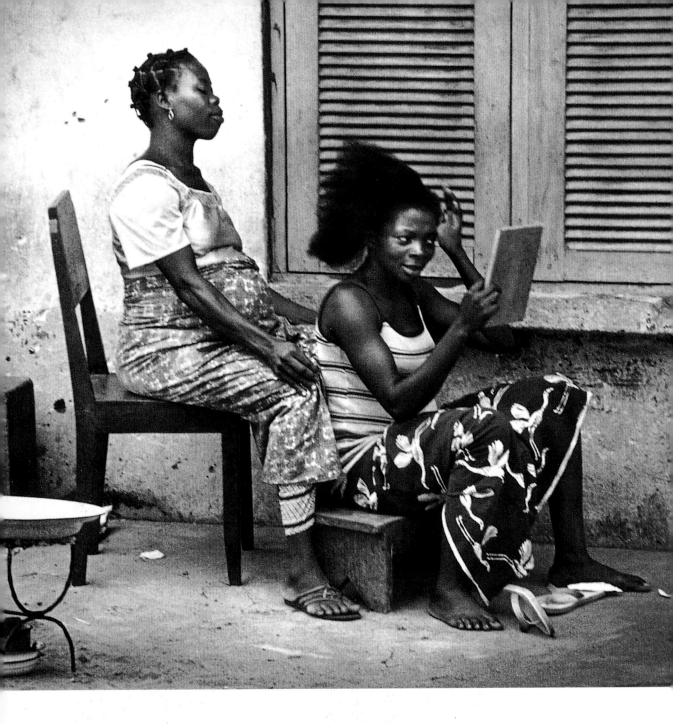

The whole experience—the ritual of dealing with hair grooming—that's pleasurable. The sitting in, everyone remembers
sitting in between some other woman's legs, having your hair
brushed and braided. The feeling of knees on your cheek.

bell hooks

. . . . the most important thing about our gas-equipped kitchen was that Mama used to do hair there. She had a "hot comb" —a fine-toothed iron instrument with a long wooden handle —and a pair of iron curlers that opened and closed like scissors: Mama would put it in the gas fire until it glowed. You could smell those prongs heating up.

I liked that smell. Not the smell so much, I guess, as what the smell meant for the shape of my day. There was an intimate warmth in the women's tones as they talked with my Mama, doing their hair. I knew what the women had been through to get their hair ready to be "done," because I would watch Mama do it to herself.

How that kink could be transformed through grease and fire into that magnificent head of wavy hair was a miracle to me. Still is.

Henry Louis Gates Jr.

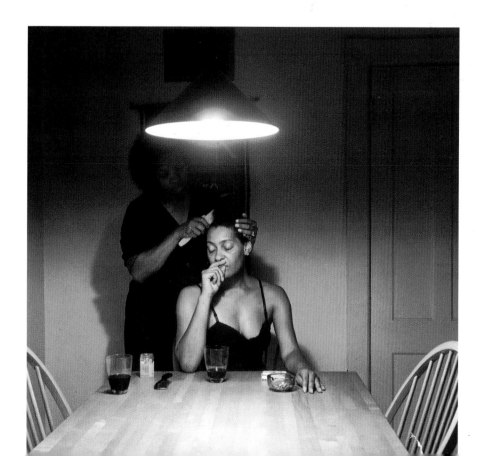

On Saturday mornings we would gather in the kitchen to get our hair fixed, that is straightened. Smells of burning grease and hair mingled with the scent of our freshly washed bodies, with collard greens cooking on the stove, with fried fish. We did not go to the hairdressers. Mama fixed our hair. Six daughters— there was no way we could have afforded hairdressers. In those days, this process of straightening black women's hair with a hot comb was not connected in my mind with the effort to look white, to live out standards of beauty set by white supremacy. It was connected solely with rites of initiation into womanhood. To arrive at that point where one's hair could be straightened was to move from being perceived as a child (whose hair could be neatly combed and braided) to being almost a woman. It was this moment of transition my sisters and I longed for.

bell hooks

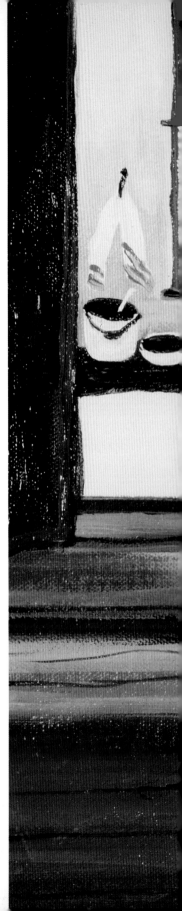

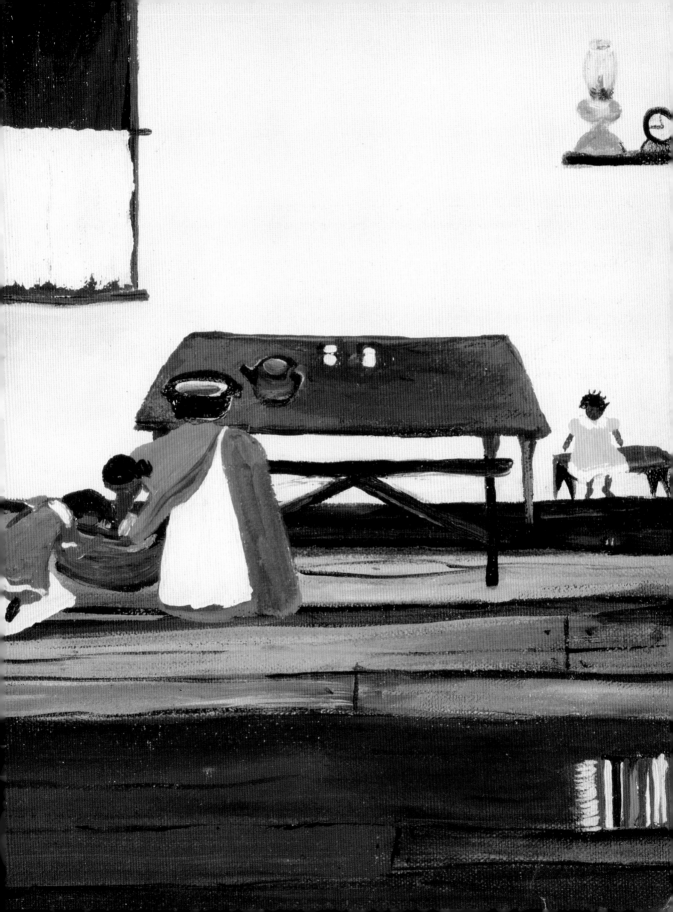

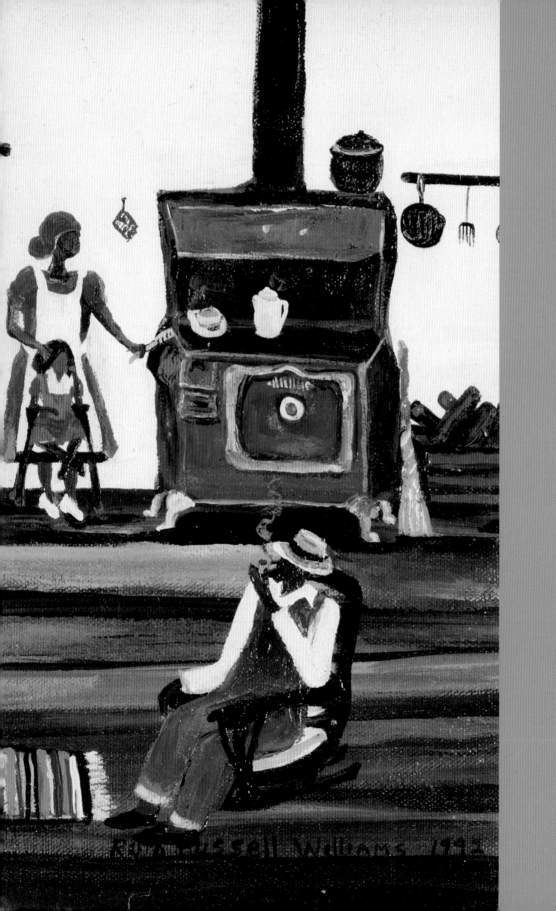

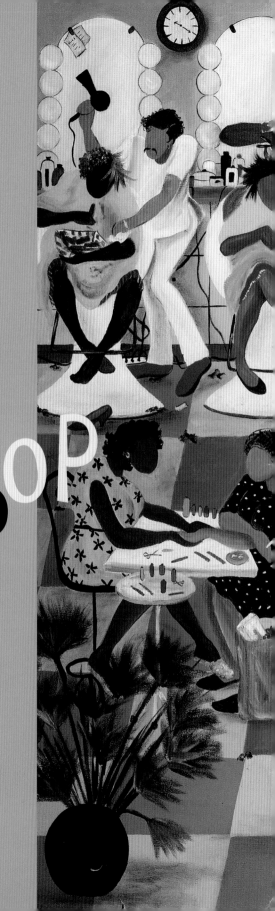

TALK TALK TALK

SHOP SHOP SHOP

Beauty parlors are
like back to your culture.
It's a meeting place,
like church.

Pauletta Lewis

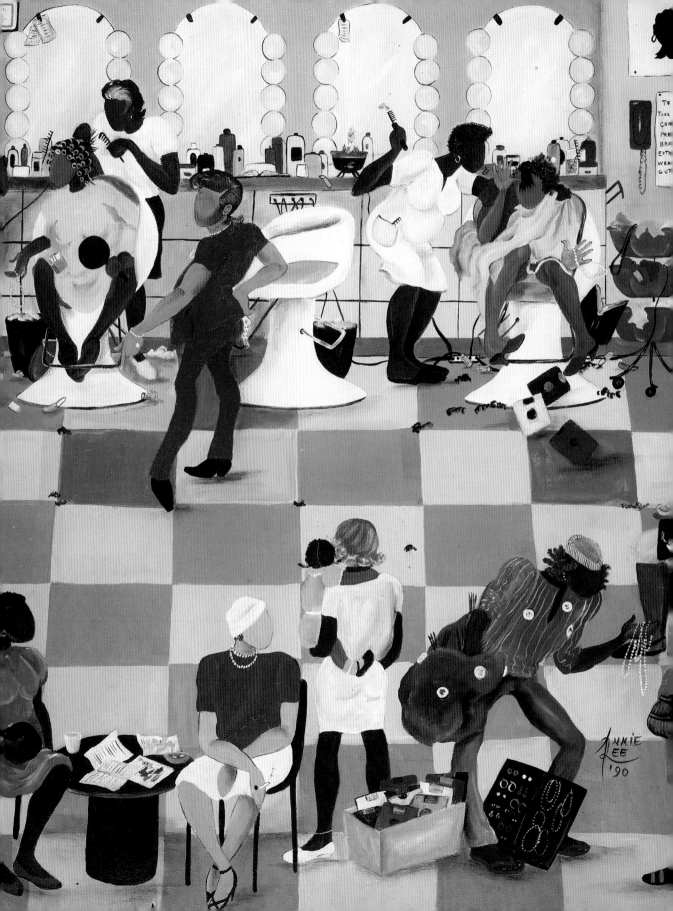

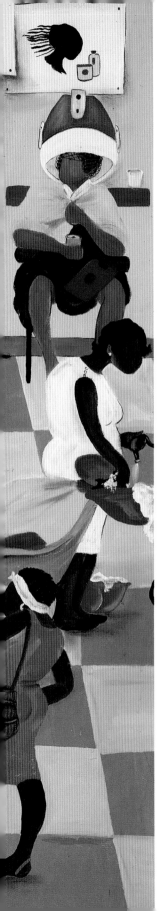

In this life there are mysteries that will never be fully understood by mere mortals.

Questions that when pondered extensively can leave the average human psyche in such a state of disarray that normal brain activity stalls, leaving the ponderer of such questions wallowing in a mass of confusion, aimlessly searching for the unknown, and ultimately leading to a state of mental chaos and cerebral shut-down. Unfortunately, as we all know, there are some questions that are better left unanswered. Questions such as

Does God really exist?

Is there life after death?

Which came first? The chicken or the egg?

Indeed, these questions can certainly leave one's mind hopelessly frazzled and disheveled. But there is an even larger question at hand today. A mystery that has eluded the genius of scholars, scientists, and political pundits alike. A question that has dogged the earth for hundreds of years, and even to this day we are nowhere near a breakthrough in this timeless riddle. The question is a serious one. The question is mind boggling.

The question is this:
Why? For the love of God!
Why does it take so long for a woman to
get her hair done at the beauty shop?

Sheneska Jackson

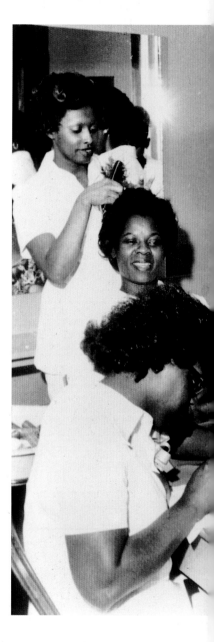

NAOLA BEAUTY ACADEMY,
NEW ORLEANS, LOUISIANA, 1943

Made Hair? The girls here
put a press on your head
last two weeks. No naps.

They learning. See the basins?
This where we wash. Yeah,
it's hot. July jam.

Stove always on. Keep the combs
hot. Lee and Ida bumping hair
right now. Best two.

Ida got a natural touch.
Don't burn nobody.
Her own's a righteous mass.

Lee, now she used to sew
Her fingers steady
from them tiny needles.

She can fix some bad hair
Look how she lay them waves.
Light, slight and polite.

Not one out of place.

Natasha Trethewey

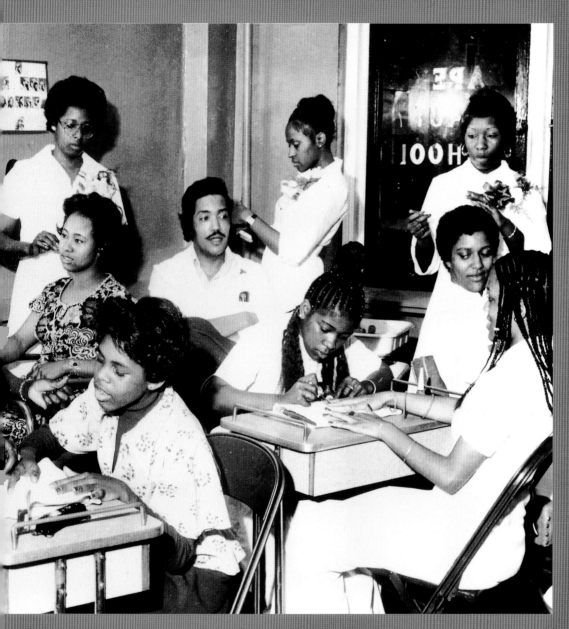

Students of Apex Beauty School
demonstrating hairstyling and
nail care, 1970s.

Just for me!

CREMA RELAJANTE SIN LEJIA

PASO 1.

PASO 2.

PASO 6.

Women's hair salons of the '30s and '40s were formal affairs, stylists wore uniforms and emphasis was placed on various techniques, or systems, as they were called, many of which incorporated hair treatments devised to address the adverse effects of hot-combing and other conditions. The image of the salon was almost like that of a glamorous doctor's clinic, designed to give women customers a sense of security and well-being in giving up care of their hair to others.

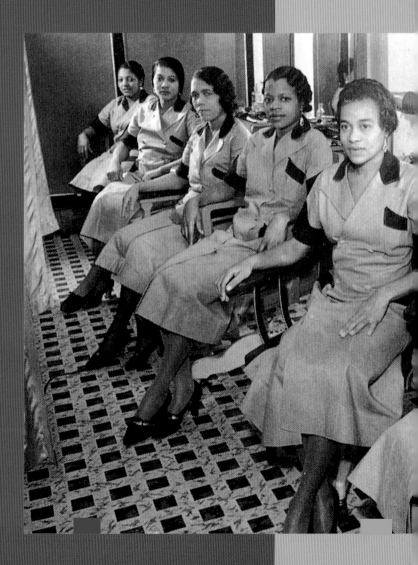

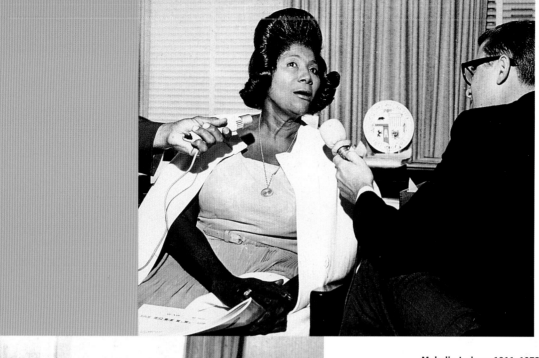

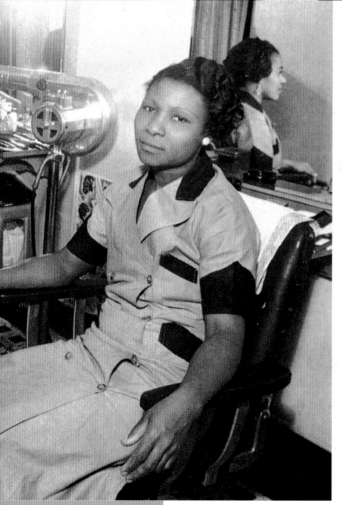

Mahalia Jackson 1911–1972

Mahalia Jackson is acknowledged as the world's greatest gospel singer. She had great presence and was often described as stately and majestic. Although her hairstyles changed several times over her career, she was best known for her sweeping updos. Her hair was a rich, jet-black sheen, pressed, rolled, sometimes finger-waved or back combed, but always styled high, which contributed in part, to her commanding presence and regal bearing. Her 1972 *New York Times*, obituary noted, "Miss Jackson was a woman on fire, whose combs flew out of her hair as she performed. She moved her listeners to dancing, to shouting, to ecstasy."

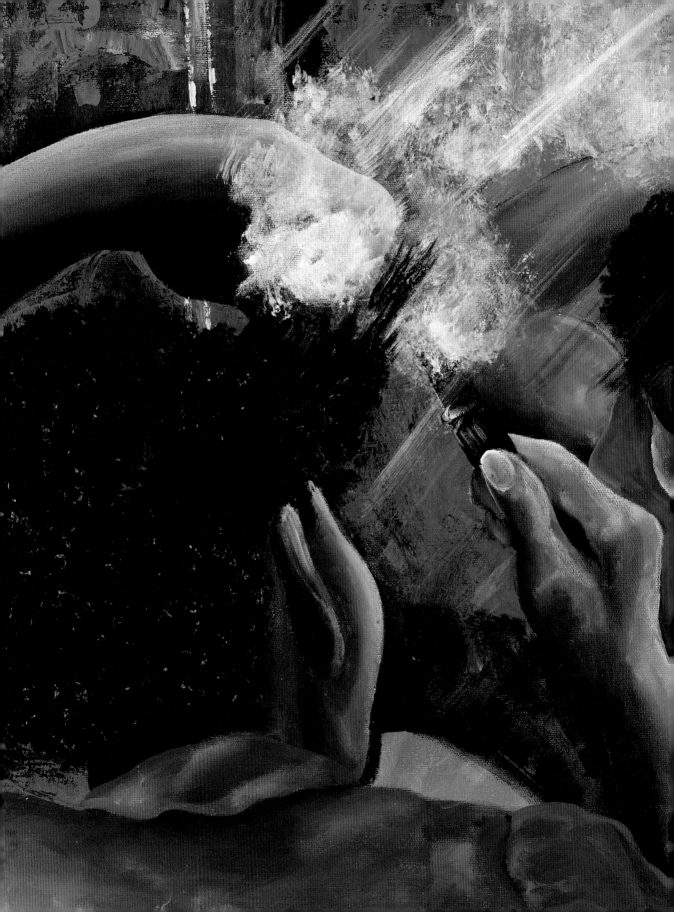

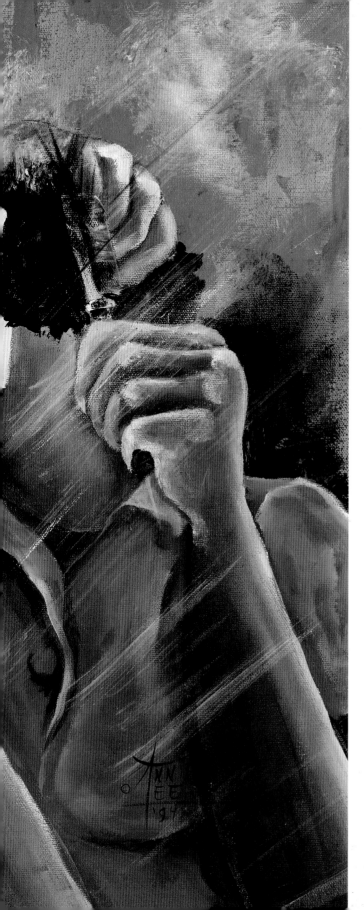

HOT COMB

Halfway through an afternoon
of coca cola bottles sweating rings
on veneered tabletops and the steel drone
of window fans above the silence
in each darkened room, I open a stiff drawer
and find the old hot combs, black
with grease, the teeth still pungent
as burning hair. One is small, fine toothed
as if for a child. Holding it,
I think of my mother's slender wrist,
the curve of her neck as she leaned over
the stove, her eyes shut as she pulled
the wooden handle and laid flat the wisps
at her temples. The heat in our kitchen
made her glow that morning I watched her
wincing, the hot comb singeing her brow,
sweat glistening above her lips,
her face made strangely beautiful
as only suffering can do.

Natasha Trethewey

AT THE HAIRDRESSERS

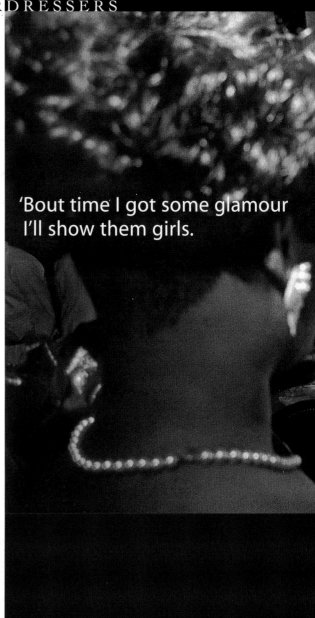

Gimme an upsweep, Minnie,
    With humpteen baby curls,

'Bout time I got some glamour
I'll show them girls.

Think they so fly a-struttin'
With they wool a-blowin' 'round.
Wait'll they see my upsweep.
That'll jop 'em back on the ground.

Got Madam C.J. Walker's first.
Got Poro Grower next.
Ain't none of 'em worked with me Min.
But I ain't vexed.

Long hair's out of style anyhow, ain't it?
Now it's tie it up high with curls.
So gimme an upsweep, Minnie.
I'll show them girls.

Gwendolyn Brooks

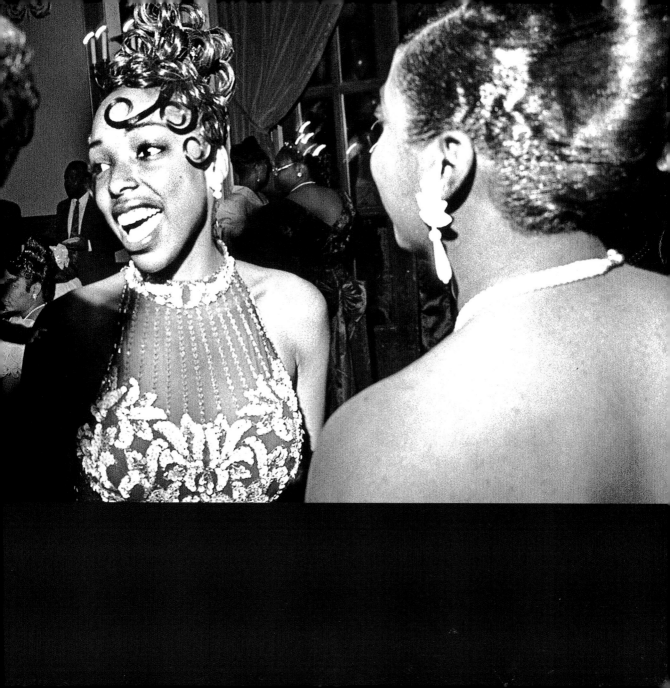

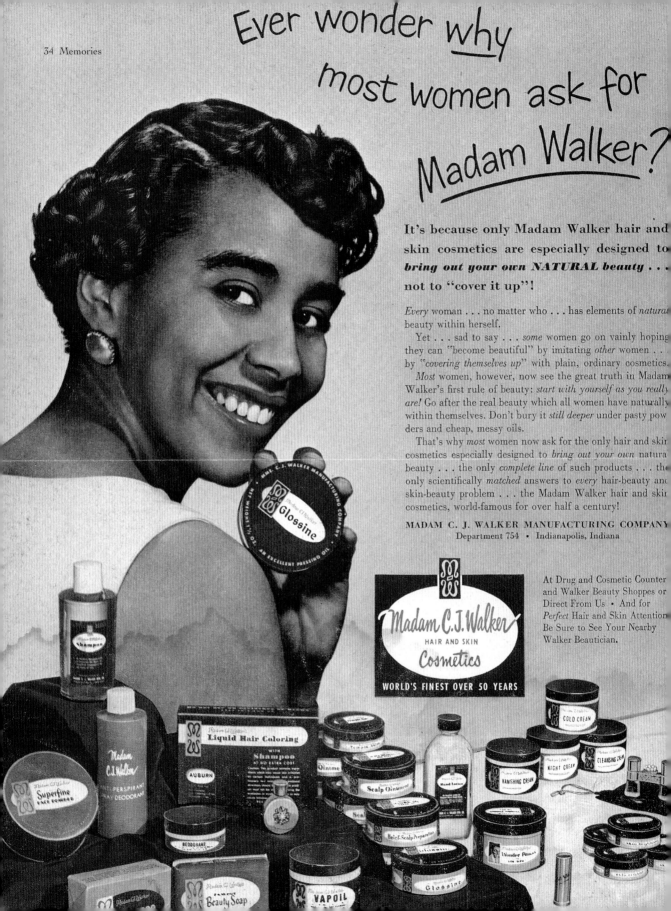

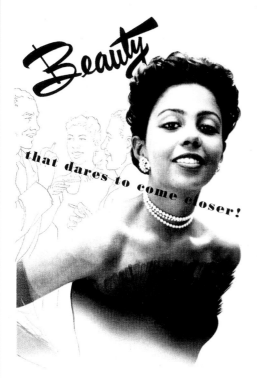

Beauty

that dares to come closer!

Only __honest beauty__ can give you __confidence!__

WHY GO ON *pretending?* Why *imitate others—in vain?* Start where Madam Walker starts: *with you as you really are!* Go after the *real* beauty which *all* women have within them. Don't bury it *still deeper* under pasty powders and messy oils.

Only Madam Walker's hair and skin cosmetics are designed to *bring out your own* natural beauty! That's why her wonderful HAIR & SCALP PREPARATION knows no rival (60¢ plus 12¢ tax) . . . why her famous GLOSSINE is the queen of all the *light-bodied* pressing oils (45¢ plus 9¢ tax) . . . why her new VAP-OIL (50¢ plus 10¢ tax) is the only *really* good way to cold-curl your hair, pressed or *unpressed,* long or short.

Don't "just *wear*" cosmetics like a hat! Buy the *best.* Discover *your own* REAL *beauty!*

Madam C. J. Walker
HAIR AND SKIN
Cosmetics
WORLD'S FINEST OVER 50 YEARS

If your dealer is temporarily "out," order direct from us. Add 20¢ on cash mail order to avoid C.O.D. costs. (Minimum C.O.D. order: $1 deposit plus postal costs). No tax if for beauty shop use, but send professional address.

MADAM C. J. WALKER MFG. CO. • DEPT. E-454 • INDIANAPOLIS, INDIANA

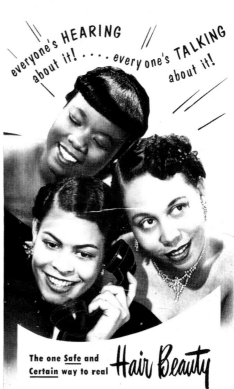

everyone's HEARING about it! . . . everyone's TALKING about it!

The one Safe and Certain way to real *Hair Beauty*

HAIR BEAUTY IS SCALP DEEP! When plain hair-dressings only cover up deep-down causes of shabby hair, it really gets worse and WORSE! BEFORE using a dressing, treat itchy or flaking scalp, dandruff or tetter with Madam Walker's DOUBLE-STRENGTH SCALP OINTMENT . . . and short, thin, brittle or falling hair by massaging scalp with HAIR & SCALP PREPARATION . . . after washing with her SHAMPOO SOAP!

THEN (NOT BEFORE) can you be sure of longest-lasting, silky-soft texture by using GLOSSINE, queen of ALL the light-bodied pressing oils and hair dressings!

BE WISE. Use your head . . . for lovely hair!

Madam C. J. Walker Mfg. Co. · Dept. 852 · Indianapolis, Ind.

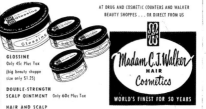

GLOSSINE Only 45¢ Plus Tax (big beauty shoppe size only $1.25)	AT DRUG AND COSMETIC COUNTERS AND WALKER BEAUTY SHOPPES . . . OR DIRECT FROM US
DOUBLE-STRENGTH SCALP OINTMENT Only 60¢ Plus Tax	**Madam C. J. Walker** HAIR *Cosmetics*
HAIR AND SCALP PREPARATION Only 60¢ Plus Tax	WORLD'S FINEST FOR 50 YEARS
TEMPLE SALVE Only 45¢ Plus Tax	FOR PERFECT HAIR ATTENTION DON'T FORGET YOUR NEARBY WALKER BEAUTICIAN!

POSTAGE PREPAID ONLY ON CASH ORDERS • NO TAX IF FOR BEAUTY SHOP USE

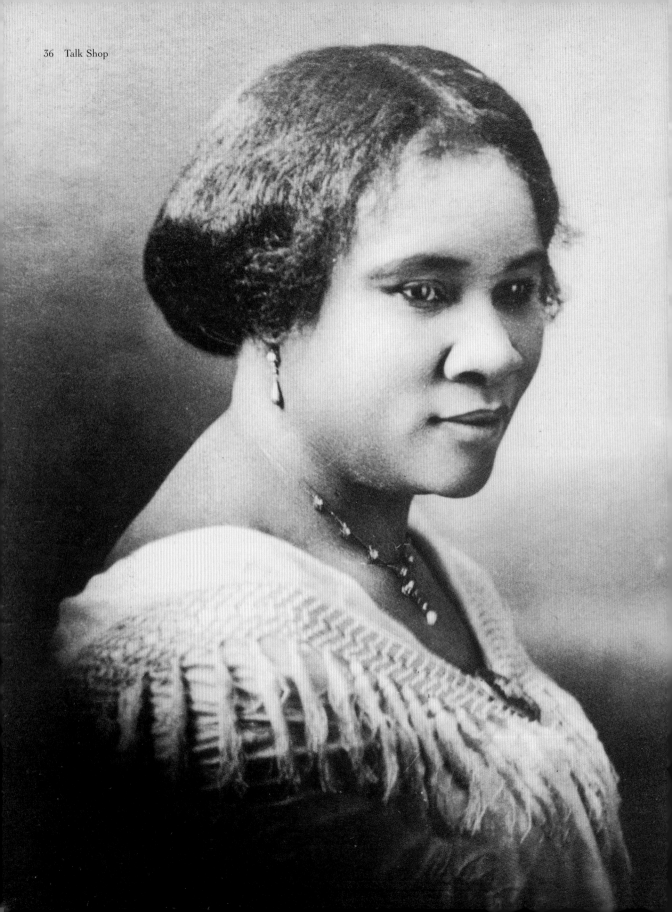

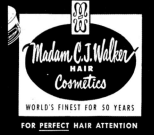

WORLD'S FINEST FOR 50 YEARS

FOR **PERFECT** HAIR ATTENTION

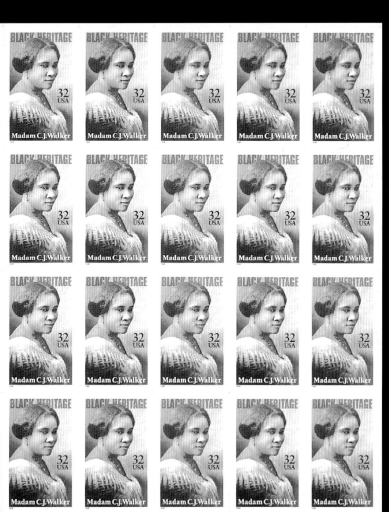

Madam C. J. Walker,
December 23, 1867–May 25, 1919. Entrepr

AMONG THE THINGS
THAT USE TO BE

Use to be
Ya could learn a whole lot of stuff
Sitting in them
beauty shop chairs

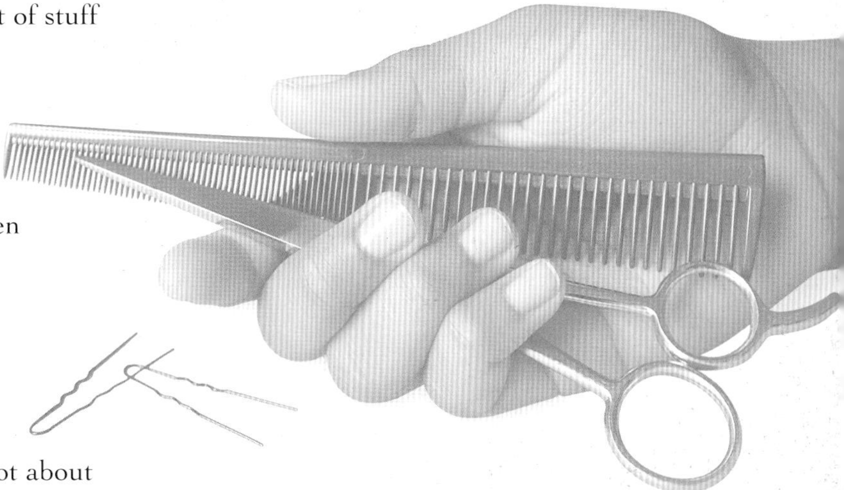

Use to be
Ya could meet
a whole lot of other women
Sittin there
along with hair frying
spit flying
and babies crying

Use to be
you could learn a whole lot about
how to catch up
with yourself
and some other folks
in your household.

Lots more got taken care of
than hair
Cause in our mutual obvious dislike
for nappiness
we came together
under the hot comb
to share
and share
and
share

But now we walk
heads high
naps full of pride
with not a backward glance
at some of the beauty which
used to be

cause with a natural
there is no natural place
For us to congregate
to mull over
our mutual discontent

Beauty shops
could have been
a hell-of-a-place
To ferment
a.........revolution.

Willi Coleman

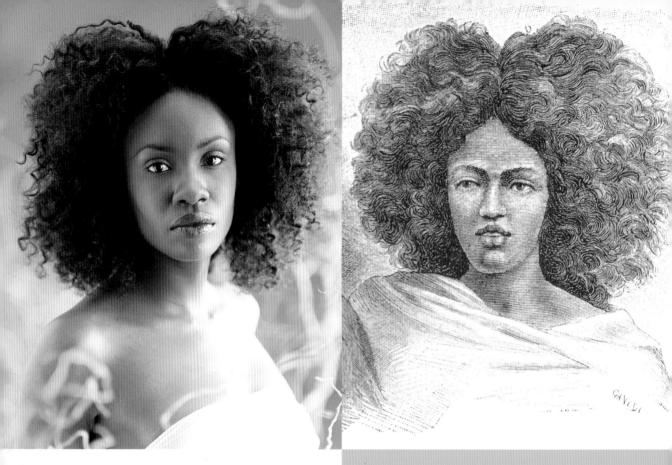

20th Century

By the end of the mid '70s, the Afro hairstyle had fallen out of fashion. It has, since then, occasionally made a comeback in the '80s and again in the late '90s with the nostalgia for retro hairstyles and fashion. The well-defined round halo associated with the Afro later on became looser, less rigid, and freer flowing.

19th Century

In many parts of Africa, hair worn loose and unstyled is considered a sign of chaos, loss of control, and even insanity. To members of the Shawan ethnic group in Ethiopia, hair worn out and uncombed is reserved for women in mourning.

19th Century

Nineteenth-century drawing of Ethiopian women's hairstyles by Guglielmo Massaia, from I miei trentacinque anni di missione nell' alta Etiopia, 1885–95.

20th Century

The echo of Africa can be in most contemporary braid styles, as we see in this spiral created out of locks, which elegantly twist upward. The spiral design is also part of this Ethiopian woman's nineteenth-century hairstyle.

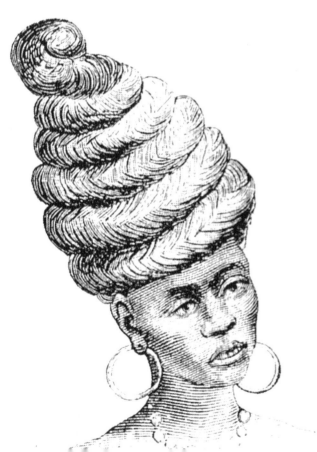

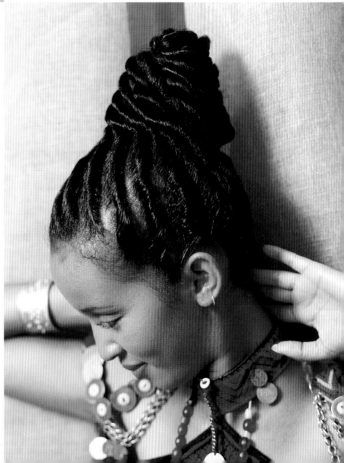

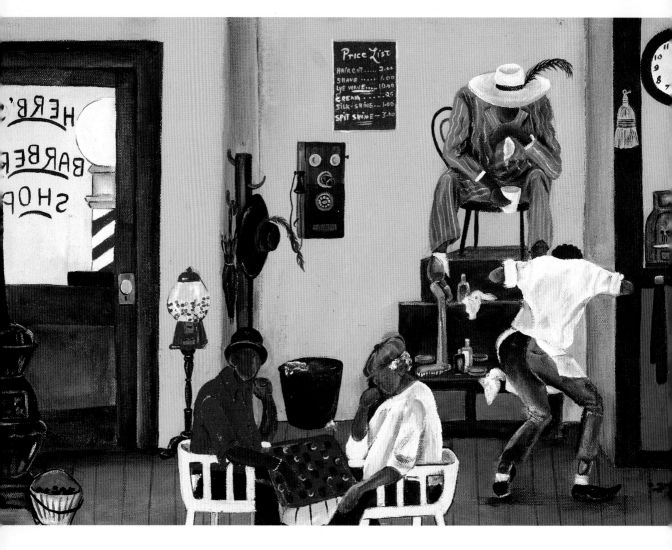

BARBERSHOP RITUAL

Baby brother can't wait.
For him, the rite of passage
begins early—before obligatory heists
of candy & comic books from neighborhood
stores, before street battles to claim
turf, before he might gain
the title "Man of the House"
before his time.

Each week, he steps up to the chair,
The closest semblance of a throne
he'll ever know, and lays in
for the cut, the counseling of
older dudes, cappin' players, men-of-words,
Greek chorus to the comic-tragic fanfare
of approaching manhood.

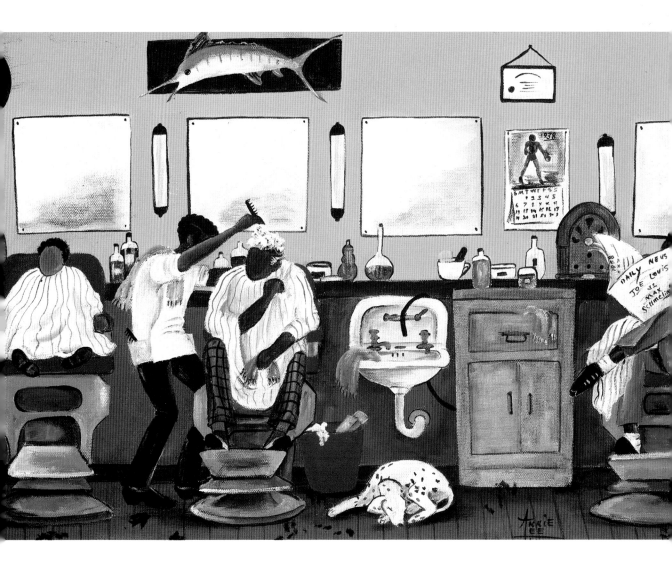

Baby brother's named for two fathers,
and each Saturday he seeks them
in this neutral zone of brotherhood,
where manhood sprouts like new growth
week by week and dark hands
deftly shape identity.

Head-bowed, church-solemn,
he sheds hair like motherlove & virginity,
weightier than Air Jordans & designer
sweats—euphemistic battle gear.
He receives the tribal standard:
a nappy helmet sporting arrows, lightning
bolts, rows of lines cut in—New World
scarification—or carved logos (Adidas,
Public Enemy) and tags, like hieroglyphic
distress signs to the ancestors:
Remember us, remember our names!

Sharan Strange

BEAUTY SHOP

Listen, ostrich plumes
differ from chicken feathers.

Okot P'Bitek,
Song of Lawino

1. Prices Subject to change without Notice
   I want my ten percent the beautician cries, her words
   quick, sharp as pink-handled cutting shears she
   uses and uses and uses on a good day. A thin hand

   on her chubby hip, she presses her license to bulletproof plastic.
   The saffron man behind it, the old man, Mister Lee, has come
   to expect her, the dollar waving droves of crusted, white gel;

   hoochies in gold, wicked clothes, Gucci-bought, fringe-trimmed,
   tight, cropped pants. A sign fading on his shop says "LeKair
   Beauty Ointment! Today On sale! Buy 16 oz. bottle. Get French Roll Free"…

   free as he mines fields of ghetto phat green,
   unfamiliar with LeKair product quotes, the way the products
   deep-skinned model in cartoon ads holds her thin hand

   to bushy frizz, says in ballooned writing "Fix This Mess"
   code for All Ways, TCB, African Pride products are not made,
   are rarely sold, by Black business.

2. Ya'll gon make me loose my mind, up in here, up in here…

   Questions from the chair on a busy Saturday

   Why, my sister, is a flat iron flat?
   Why is Lil' Kim basted in out cold gold?
   Home Girl!! Whazz UP!!! Ya better watch my ear!
   Why is my scalp sizzling? Making noises?
   Why do Black women wear yak on their heads?
   Why is "French Refined" wavy or kinky straight?
   Why does 100% human hair come only from Asia?
   Why is my hair, your hair, the old money it makes,
   territory in our community to be conquered?

Karen Williams

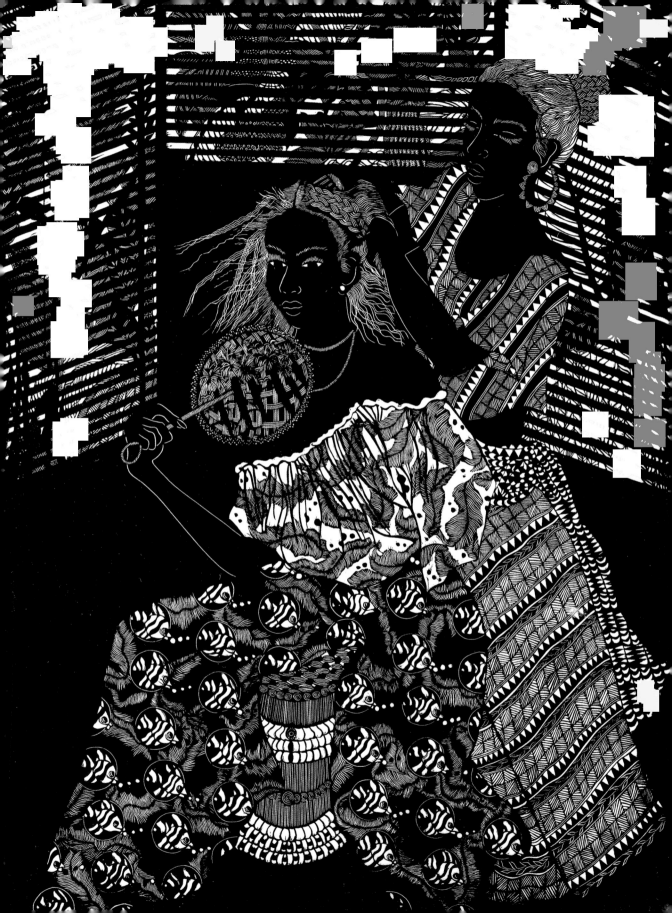

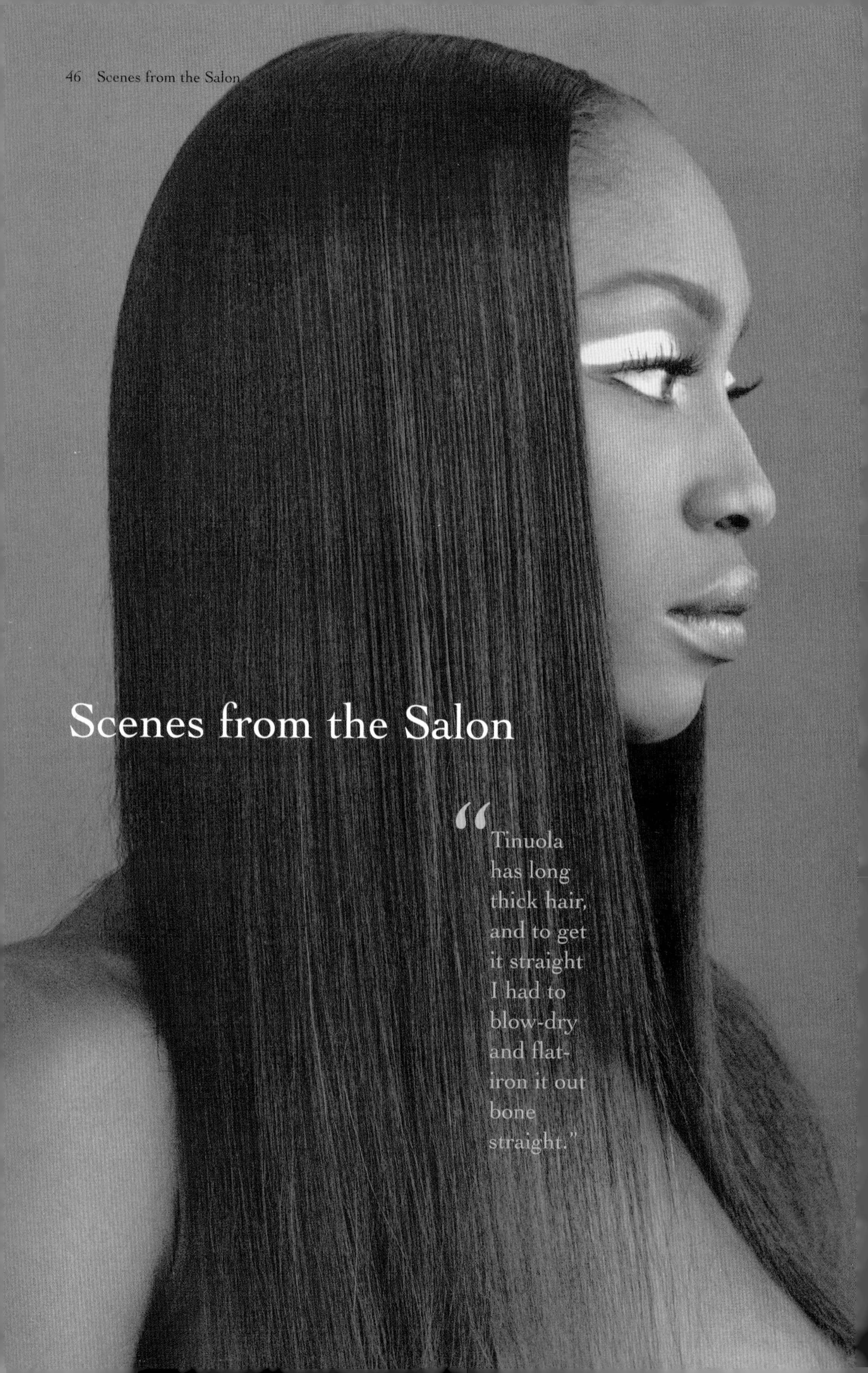

Scenes from the Salon

"Tinuola
has long
thick hair,
and to get
it straight
I had to
blow-dry
and flat-
iron it out
bone
straight."

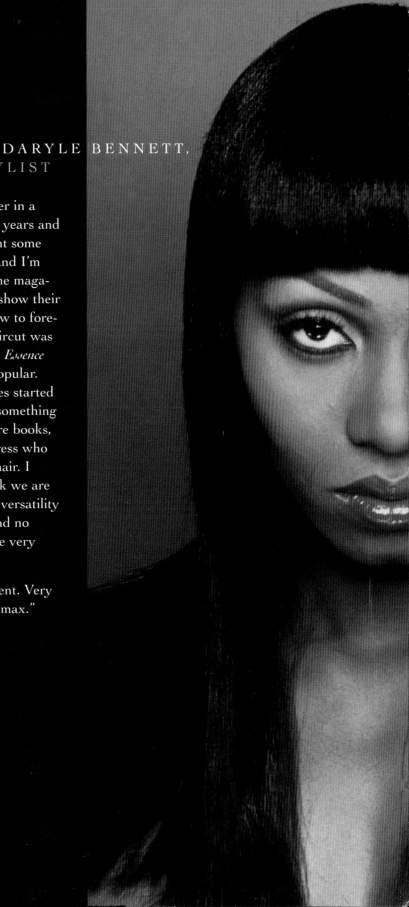

DARYLE BENNETT,
HAIR STYLIST

"I started fifteen years ago as a barber in a
barbershop. I worked there for two years and
then opened up my own salon. I sent some
pictures to *Essence* they liked them and I'm
still doing shoots for them today. The magazine is an outlet for black artists to show their
talent and to show black women how to fore-
cast new looks. The Halle Berry haircut was
one of those new looks where when *Essence*
showed it, it immediately became popular.
Every hairstylist in the United States started
doing Halle Berry haircuts. It was something
everyone had to have. We need more books,
TV shows, and magazines that express who
we are and how we feel about our hair. I
think the variety is good. I just think we are
beautiful people, and we have such versatility
with our hair. We can wear it all, and no
one else can do that. We ought to be very
proud of that."

"Working for models is a little different. Very
often you can take hairstyles to the max."

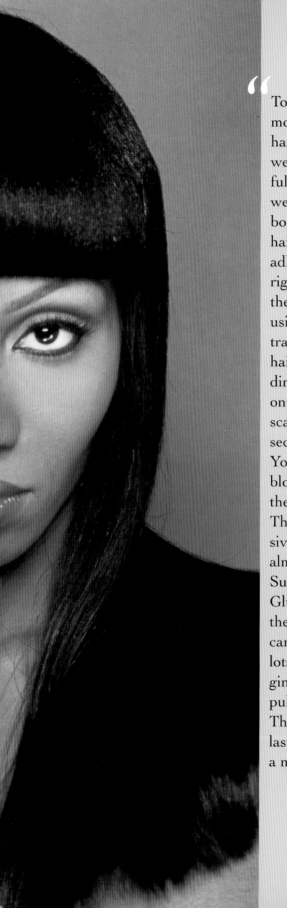

"To get the model's hair long we put in a full-head weave. We bonded her hair with adhesive right onto the scalp using tracks of hair placed directly onto the scalp by section. You then blow-dry the hair. The adhesive is almost like Super Glue, and the hair can stand lots of tugging and pulling. The style lasts about a month."

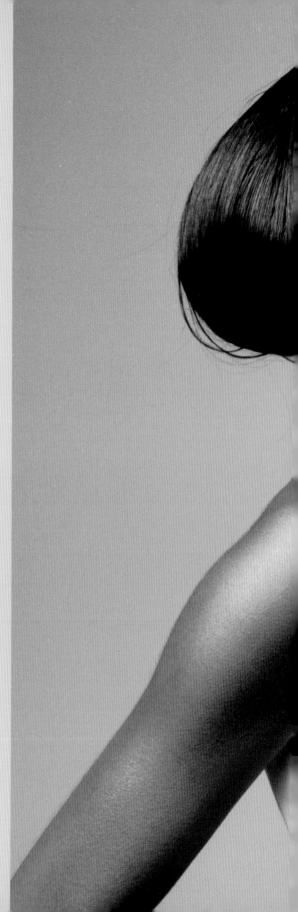

"Here we wanted something a little out of the ordinary, something very editorial and funky. I curled and shaped the entire hair. It took a lot of pins and a lot of spray to get this look."

We attached big round balls to each side of the head underneath and then combed the top layer over each ball. It took a lot of teasing and shaping of the hair. It was fantastic, I really enjoyed creating it.

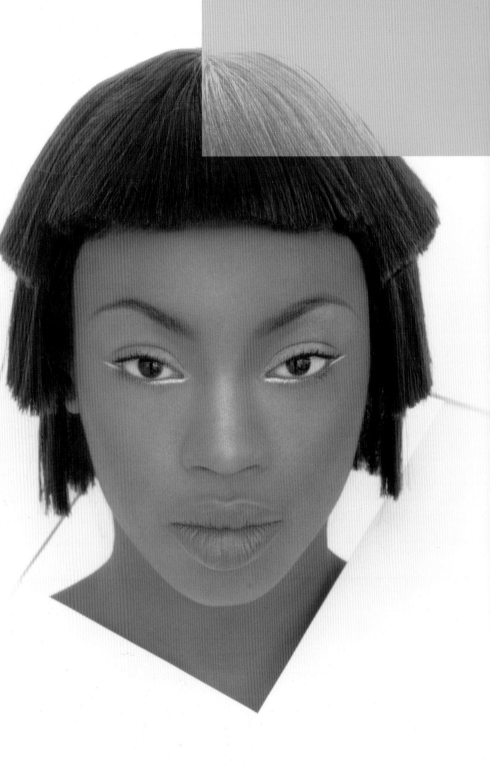

" This is a tri-level cut; it's a very archi-tectural style.

The hair was bonded on giving the model a full length of hair. I then made even parts all the way around to the level I wanted it. I cut the first bottom layer, then measured about two inches up, and cut the second layer and then the third.**"**

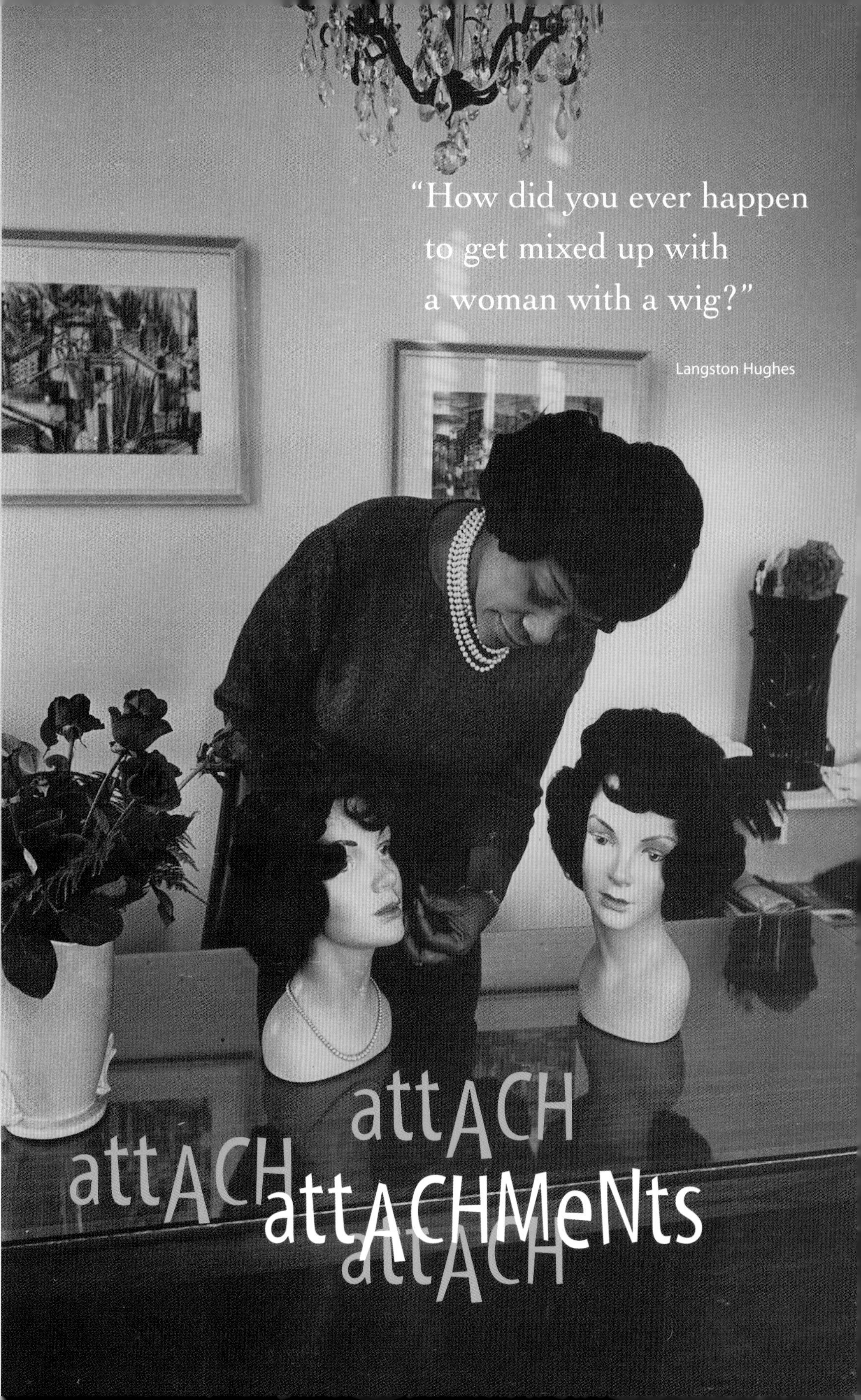

"How did you ever happen
to get mixed up with
a woman with a wig?"

Langston Hughes

attACH
attACH
attACHMeNts
attACH

The hair decoration beloved by Mauritanian women is to be seen in its most sumptuous and varied forms among the Guedra dancers. Every plait is embellished with pendants, carved shell discs called *el bot min teffou,* and triangular talismans, khourb (of green and red glass), and carnelian. Hairstyles vary from one area of Mauritania to another and within different social groups.

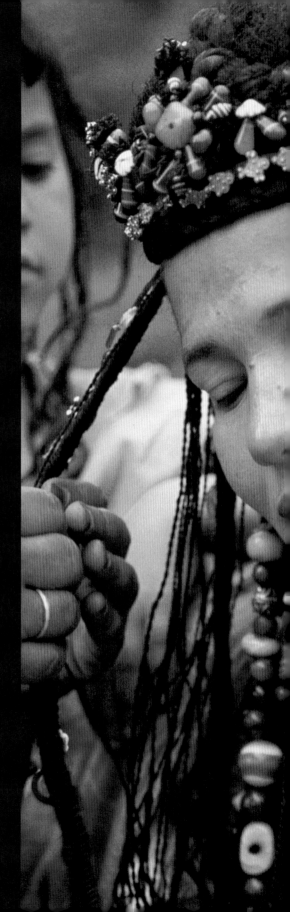

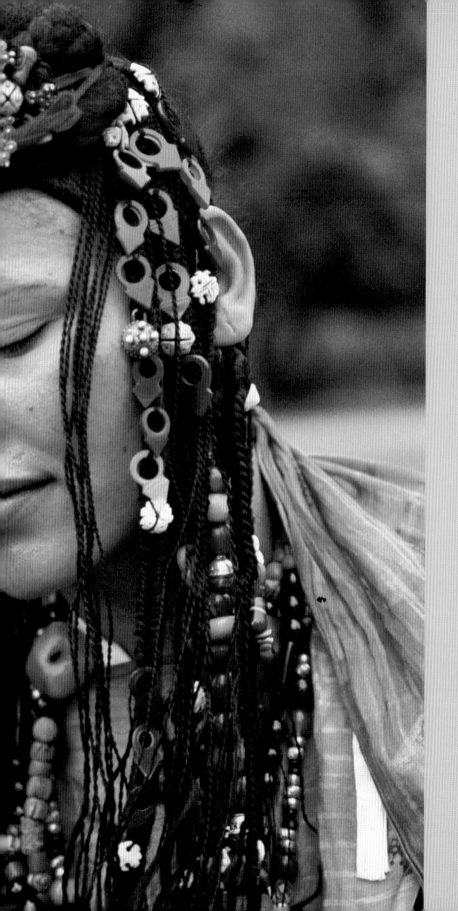

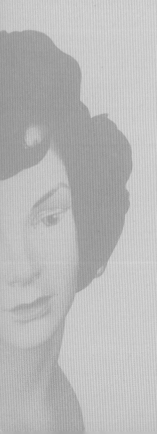

THE HAIRPIECE

As "Respect" fades into the background, a vanity revolves to center stage. On this vanity are two wigs, an Afro wig, circa 1968, and a long, flowing wig, both resting on wig stands. A black WOMAN enters, her head and body wrapped in towels. She picks up a framed picture and after a few moments of hesitation, throws it into a small trash can. She then removes one of her towels to reveal a totally bald head. Looking into a mirror of the "fourth wall," she begins applying makeup.

The wig stand holding the Afro wig opens her eyes. Her mame is JANINE. She stares in disbelief at the bald woman.

JANINE:
(Calling to the other wig stand)
La Wanda.
La Wanda girl, wake up.

LAWANDA:
What? What is it?

JANINE:
Check out girlfriend.

LAWANDA:
Oh, girl, I don't believe it.

JANINE: (Laughing.)
Just look at the poor thing, trying to paint some life onto that face of hers. You'd think by now she'd realize it's the hair. It's all about the hair.

LAWANDA:
What hair! She ain't go no hair! She done fried, dyed, de-chemicalized her shit to death.

JANINE:
And, all that's left is that buck-naked scalp of hers, sittin' up there apologizin' for being odd-shaped and ugly.

LAWANDA: (Laughing with JANINE)
Girl, stop!

JANINE:
I ain't sayin' nuthin' but the truth.

LAWANDA/JANINE:

The bitch is bald!

They laugh.

JANINE:
And all over some man.

LAWANDA:
I tell ya, girl, I just don't understand it. I mean, look at her. She's got a right nice face, a good head on her shoulders. A good job even. And she's got to go fall in love with that fool.

JANINE:
That political quick-change artist. Everytime the nigga went and changed his ideology, she went and changed her hair to fit the occasion.

LAWANDA:
Well at least she's breaking up with him.

JANINE:
Hunny, no!

LAWANDA:
Yes child.

JANINE:
Oh, girl, dish me the dirt!

LAWANDA:
Well, you see, I heard her on the phone talking to one of her girlfriends, and she's meeting him for lunch today to give him the ax.

JANINE:
Well it's about time.

LAWANDA:
I hear ya. But don't you worry 'bout a thing, girlfriend. I'm gonna tell you all about it.

JANINE:
Hunny, you won't have to tell me a damn thing 'cause I'm gonna be there, front row, center.

LAWANDA:
You?

JANINE:
Yes child, she's wearing me to lunch.

LAWANDA: (Outraged.)
I don't think so!

JANINE: (With an attitude.)
What do you mean, you don't think so?

LAWANDA:
Exactly what I said, "I don't think so."
Damn, Janine, get real. How the hell she gonna wear both of us?

JANINE:

She ain't wearing both of us. She's wearing me.

LAWANDA:

Says who?

JANINE:
Says me! Says her!
Ain't that right, girlfriend?

The WOMAN stops putting on her makeup, looks around, sees no one, and goes back to her makeup.

JANINE:
I said, ain't that right!

The WOMAN picks up the phone.

WOMAN: Hello . . . hello . . .

JANINE:
Did you hear the damn phone ring?

WOMAN: No

JANINE:
Then put the damn phone down and talk to me.

WOMAN: I ah . . . don't understand.

JANINE:
It ain't deep so don't panic. Now you're having lunch with your boyfriend, right?

WOMAN: (Breaking into tears)
I think I'm having a nervous breakdown.

JANINE: (Impatient)
I said you're having lunch with your boyfriend, right!

WOMAN: (Scared, pulling herself together)
Yes, right . . . right.

JANINE:
To break up with him.

WOMAN:
How did you know that?

LAWANDA:
I told her.

WOMAN: (Stands and screams)
Help! Help!

JANINE:
Sit down. I said sit your ass down!

The WOMAN does.

JANINE:
Now set her straight and tell her you're wearing me.

LAWANDA:
She's the one who needs to be set straight, so go on and tell her you're wearing me.

JANINE:
No, tell her you're wearing me.

There is a pause.

LAWANDA:
Well?

JANINE:
Well?

WOMAN:

I ah . . . actually hadn't made up my mind.

JANINE: (Going off)
What do you mean you ain't made up your mind! After all that fool has put you through, you gonna need all the attitude you can get, and there is nothing like attitude and a healthy head of kinks to make his shit shrivel like it should!

That's right! When you wearin' me, you lettin' him know he ain't gonna get no sweet-talkin' comb through your love without some serious resistance. No-no! The kink of my head is like the king of your heart, and neither is about to be hot-pressed into surrender.

LAWANDA:
That shit is so tired. The last time attitude worked on anybody was 1968. Janine, girl, you need to get over it and get on with it. (To the WOMAN) And you need to give the nigga a good-bye he will never forget.

I say give him hysteria! Give him emotion! Give him rage! And there is nothing like a toss of the tresses to make your emotional outburst shine with emotional flair.

You can toss me back, shake me from side to side, all the while screaming, "I want you out of my life forever!!!" And not only will I come bouncing back for more, but you just might win an Academy Award for best performance by a head of hair in a dramatic role.

JANINE:

Miss hunny, please! She don't need no Barbie doll dipped in chocolate telling her what to do. She needs a head of hair that's coming from a fo' real place.

LAWANDA:

Don't you dare talk about nobody coming from a "fo' real place," Miss Made-in-Taiwan!

JANINE:

Hey! I ain't ashamed of where I come from. Besides, it don't matter where you come from as long as you end up in the right place.

LAWANDA:

And it don't matter the grade as long as the point gets made. So go on and tell her you're wearing me.

JANINE:

No, tell her you're wearing me.

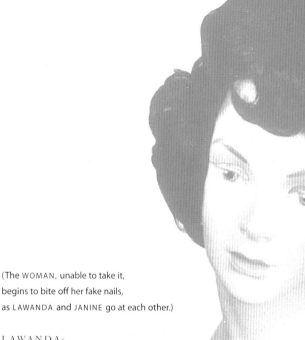

(The WOMAN, unable to take it, begins to bite off her fake nails, as LAWANDA and JANINE go at each other.)

LAWANDA:

Set the bitch straight. Let her know there is no way she could even begin to compete with me.

I am quality. She is kink. I am exotic. She is common. I am class, and she is trash. That's right. T.R.A.S.H.

We're talking three strikes and you're out. So go on and tell her you're wearing me. Go on, tell her! Tell her! Tell her!

JANINE:

Who you callin' a bitch? Why, if I had hands I'd knock you clear into next week. You think you cute. She thinks she's cute just 'cause that synthetic mop of hers blows in the wind. She looks like a fool, and you look like an even bigger fool when you wear her, so go on and tell her you're wearing me. Go on, tell her! Tell her! Tell her!

(The WOMAN screams and pulls the two wigs off the wig stands as the lights go to black on three bald heads.)

George C. Wolfe

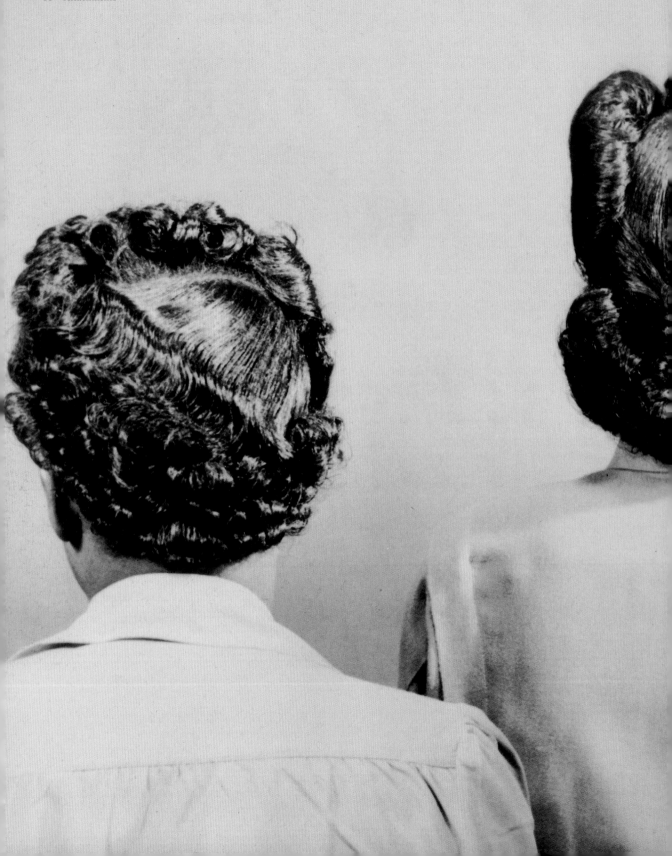

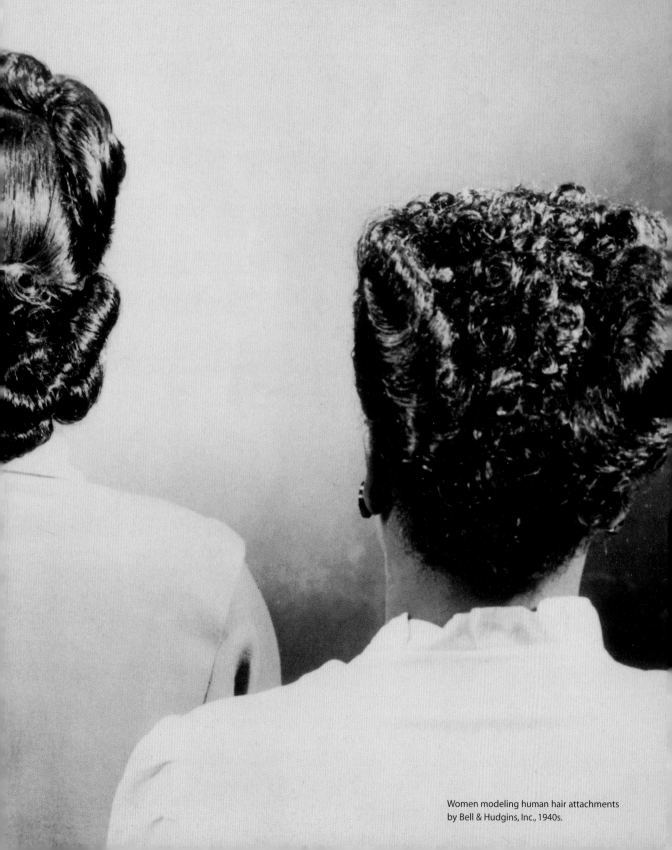

Women modeling human hair attachments
by Bell & Hudgins, Inc., 1940s.

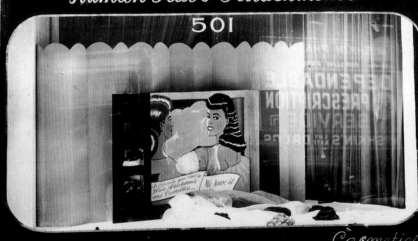

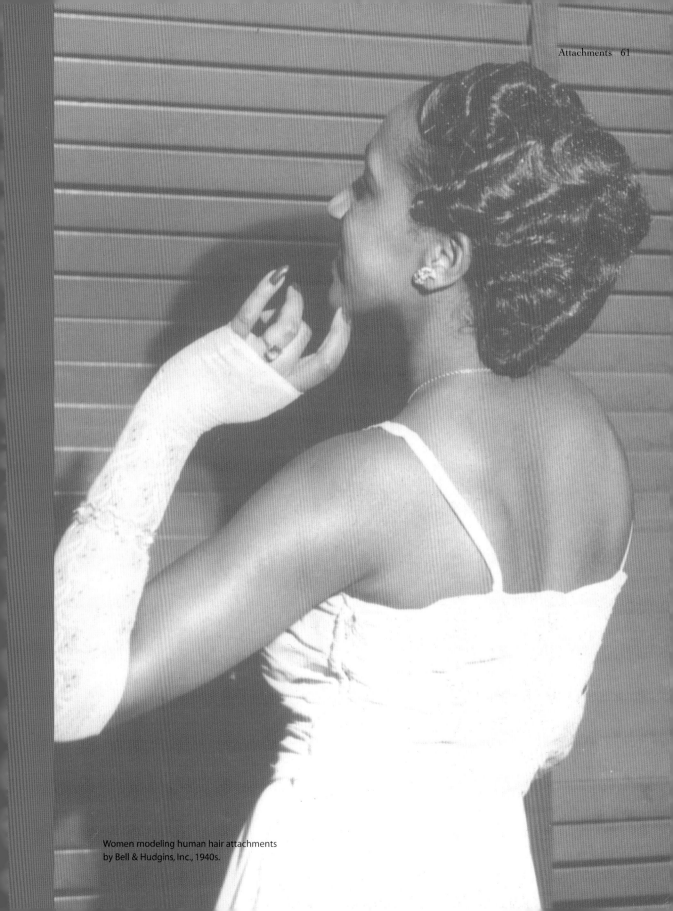

Women modeling human hair attachments
by Bell & Hudgins, Inc., 1940s.

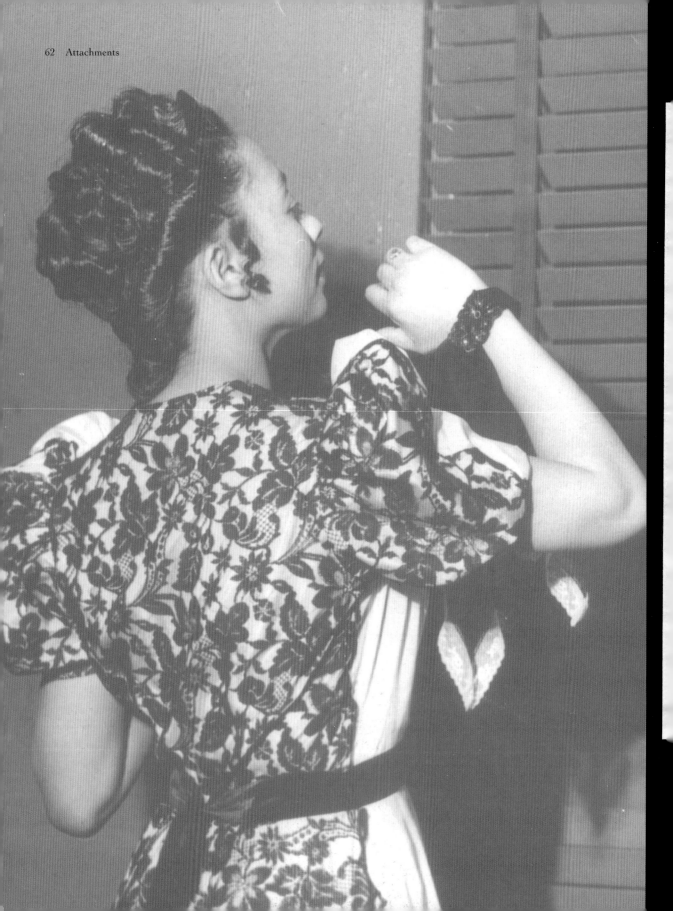

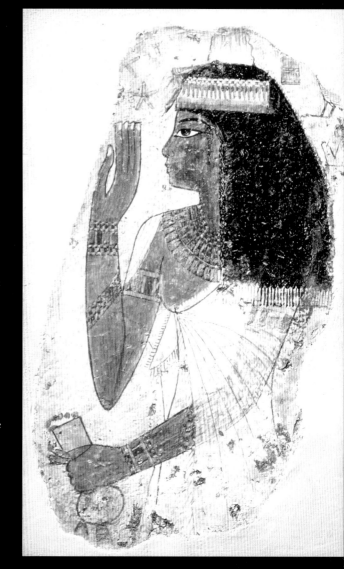

Ancient Egypt was one of the earliest societies we know of in which beauty was important. The archaeological evidence is very good here. Paintings, combs, hairpins, wigs, and romantic poetry all reveal the importance of hair for the ancient Egyptians.

The ancient Egyptians thought thick hair was best, and they liked elaborate hairstyles. They used hair extensions and wigs made of real hair, horsehair, palm-leaves, straw, or sheep's wool. The wigs were usually divided into three sections with one going down the back and two down either side at the front to the breasts. They even dyed their hair and wigs a variety of colors with blues, greens, blonds, and gold being among the preferred colors. Though black wigs hued by indigo were the favorite. It was also believed that a woman's wig could enhance her sexuality. Men also wore wigs, which although smaller than a woman's, were often more complex in design. Wigs were often scented with perfume, and wealthy Egyptians had personal barbers.

Michael Sones

WIGS, WOMEN, AND FALSIES

"I wonder why peoples, when they haven their pictures taken, always take their face? Some womens," said Simple, "have much better looking parts elsewhere.

"You can pose the doggonedest questions," I said.

"Another thing I would like to know is why people's eyebrows do not grow longer, like their hair?" asked Simple.

"I do not know,"
I answered.

"But, come to think of it," said Simple, "some people's hair on their heads don't grow no longer than their eyebrows. In fact, some women's hair don't hardly grow an inch. Yet most mens have to go to the barbershop every two or three weeks. It should be men's hair that won't grow, not the women's. Why is that?"

"I am not a student of human hair, man, so I cannot tell."

"I knowed a girl once who was too lazy to comb her head," said Simple, "so she bought herself a wig. But she was too lazy to comb that. She would just put it on her head like a hat, and go on down the street."

"You have certainly known some strange people," I said.

"I have, daddy-o, but I have never seen nothing worse than a wet wig," said Simple.

"A wet wig?" I asked. "Where on earth did you ever see a wet wig?"

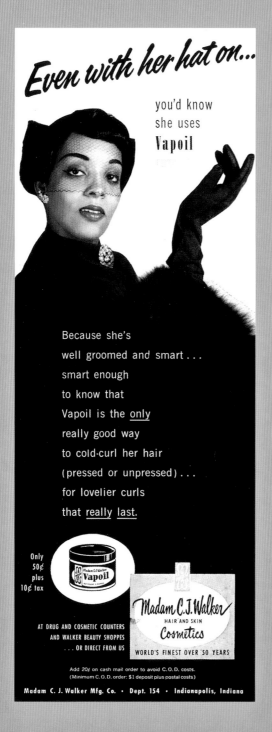

Even with her hat on...

you'd know
she uses
Vapoil

Because she's

well groomed and smart . . .

smart enough

to know that

Vapoil is the only

really good way

to cold-curl her hair

(pressed or unpressed) . . .

for lovelier curls

that really last.

Only
50¢
plus
10¢ tax

Vapoil

Madam C.J. Walker
HAIR AND SKIN
Cosmetics
WORLD'S FINEST OVER 50 YEARS

AT DRUG AND COSMETIC COUNTERS
AND WALKER BEAUTY SHOPPES
. . . OR DIRECT FROM US

Add 20¢ on cash mail order to avoid C.O.D. costs.
(Minimum C.O.D. order: $1 deposit plus postal costs.)

Madam C. J. Walker Mfg. Co. • Dept. 154 • Indianapolis, Indiana

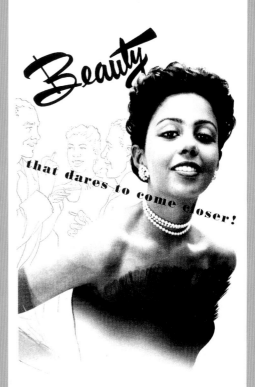

Beauty

that dares to come closer!

**Only honest beauty
can give you confidence!**

WHY GO ON *pretending?* Why *imitate others—in vain?*
Start where Madam Walker starts: *with you as you
really are!* Go after the *real* beauty which *all* women
have within them. Don't bury it *still deeper*
under pasty powders and messy oils.

Only Madam Walker's hair and skin cosmetics are
designed to *bring out your own* natural beauty!
That's why her wonderful HAIR & SCALP PREPARATION
knows no rival (60¢ plus 12¢ tax) . . . why her famous
GLOSSINE is the queen of all the *light-bodied*
pressing oils (45¢ plus 9¢ tax) . . . why her new
VAPOIL (50¢ plus 10¢ tax) is the only *really good*
way to cold-curl your hair, pressed *or unpressed,*
long or short.

Don't "just *wear*" cosmetics like a hat! Buy the *best.*
Discover *your own* REAL *beauty!*

Madam C.J. Walker
HAIR AND SKIN
Cosmetics
WORLD'S FINEST OVER 50 YEARS

If your dealer is temporarily "out,"
order direct from us. Add 20¢ on cash
mail order to avoid C.O.D. costs. (Minimum C.O.D. order: $1 deposit plus
postal costs). No tax if for beauty shop
use, but send professional address.

MADAM C. J. WALKER MFG. CO. • DEPT. E-454 • INDIANAPOLIS, INDIANA

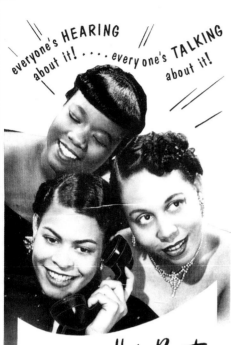
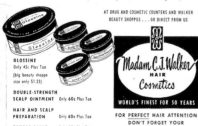
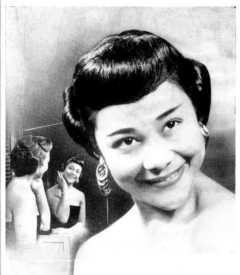

"On the beach," said Simple. "I seed a girl lose her wig in the water out at Coney Island. That woman had no business diving under the waves when she were in swimming, but she did. And off come her wig, which started riding the waves its own self. That girl were so embarrassed that she would not come out of the water until the lifeguard rowed out in a boat and got her wig, which, by that time, were headed for the open sea. She slapped the wig on her head. But it were a sight, tangled up like a hurrah's nest, and dripping like a wet dishrag. I never did see that woman go in swimming no more. In fact, I never took her to the beach again."

"How did you ever happen to get mixed up with a woman with a wig?" I asked.

"There is no telling who a man might get mixed up with at times," said Simple, "because in them days I were you and simple myself. Besides, she did not call it a wig. She called it a 'transformation.'

I do not know why they call wigs 'transformations,' because I have seen some womens put on a wig and they were not transformed at all. Now, what I would recommend to some womens is that they get wigs for their faces—which, in some cases, needs to be hidden more than their heads. Some womens is homely, Jack! So if they gonna transform themselves, they ought to start in front instead of in the back."

"Some do," I said, "with falsies."

"Don't mention falsies to me," said Simple. "It's getting so
nobody can tell how a woman is shaped any more, because
they takes their shapes off when they get home. All those
New Forms and Maiden Bras and Foam Rubber Sillhouettes!
I think there ought to be a law!

"That would be a bit drastic," I said.

"Don't you believe women have the right
to make themselves more attractive?
A little artifice here and there — lipstick,
rouge, transformations, and such."

"And such too much is what some of them does," said Simple.
"A wigless woman without her lipstick, rouge, and falsies would
be another person. Impersonating herself, that's what! If it is
wrong for a Negro to pass for white, it ought also to be wrong
for any woman to pass for what she is not. Am not I right?"

"Every woman wants to put her best face forward," I said,
"especially when she's out in public. At home, that's another
matter. And you don't go home with every woman you see."

"I might try if my jive works," said Simple.

"You'd let yourself in for some rude shocks," I said.

"A man takes a chance these days and times," said Simple.
"But then, men was born to take chances."

Langston Hughes

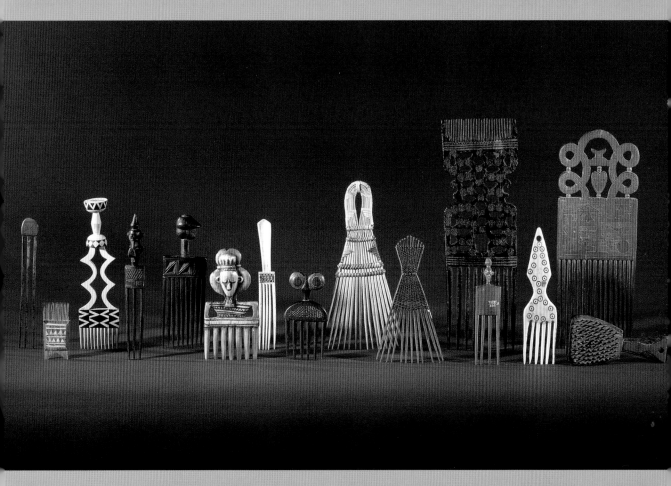

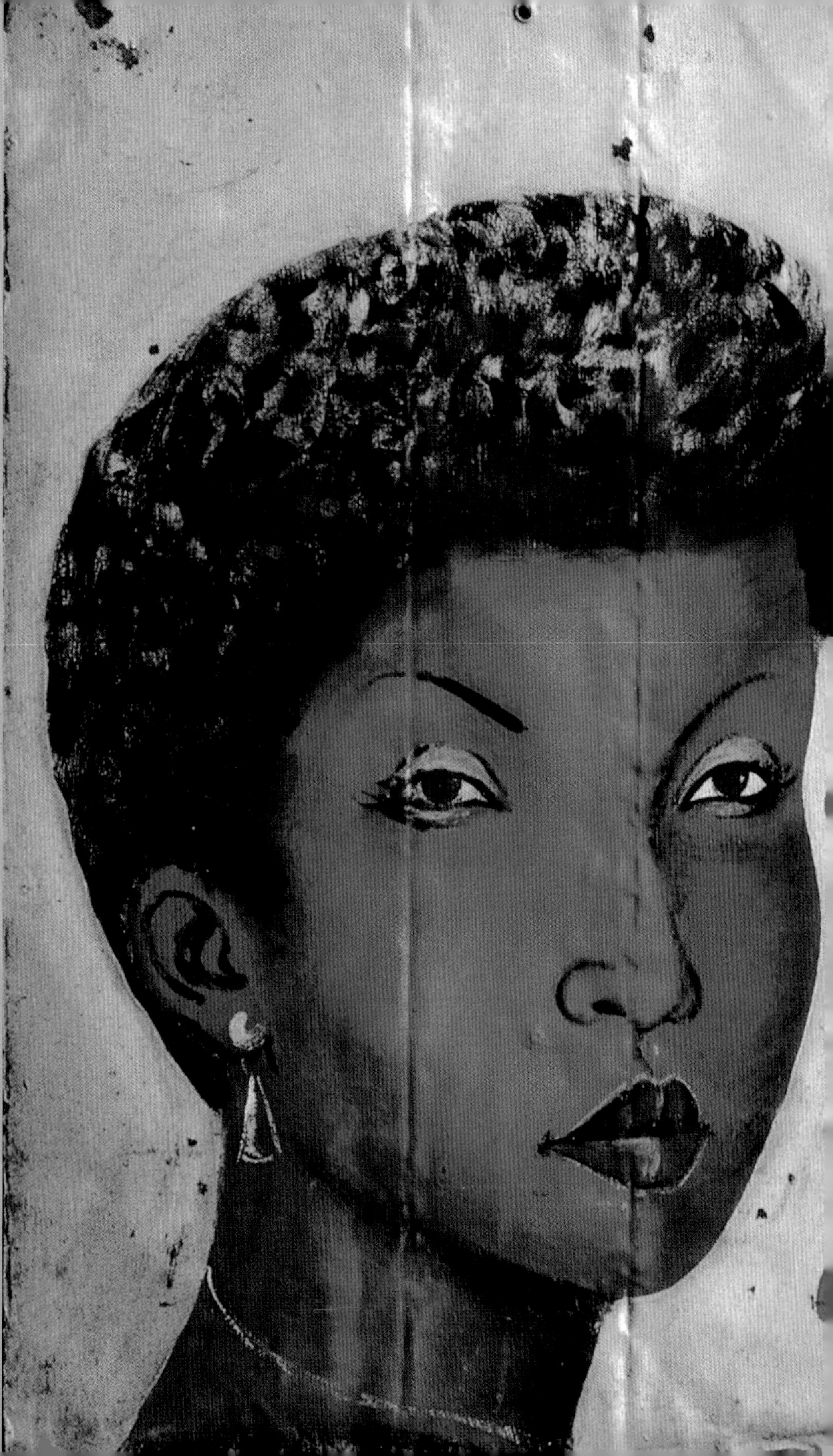

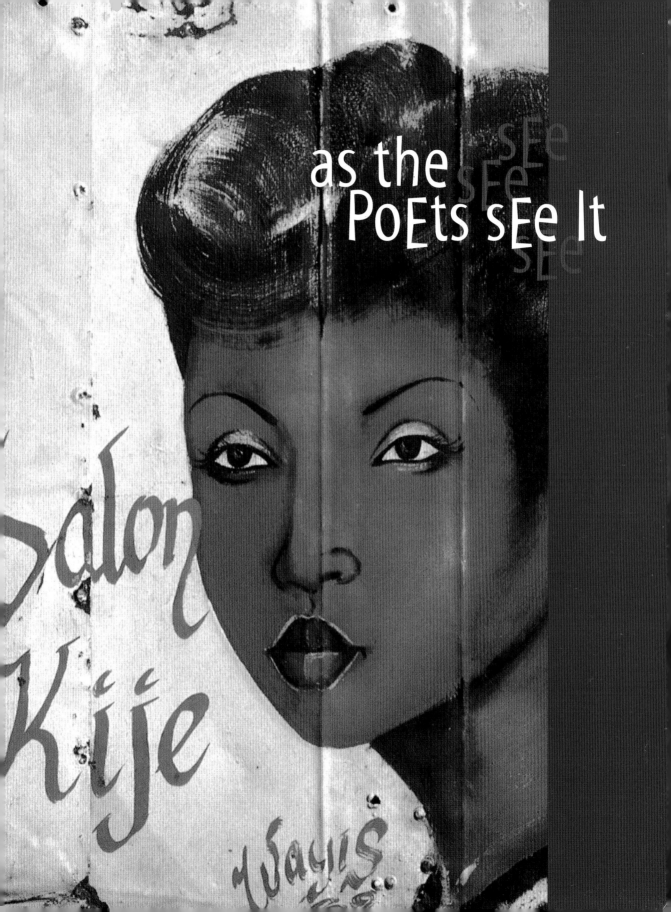

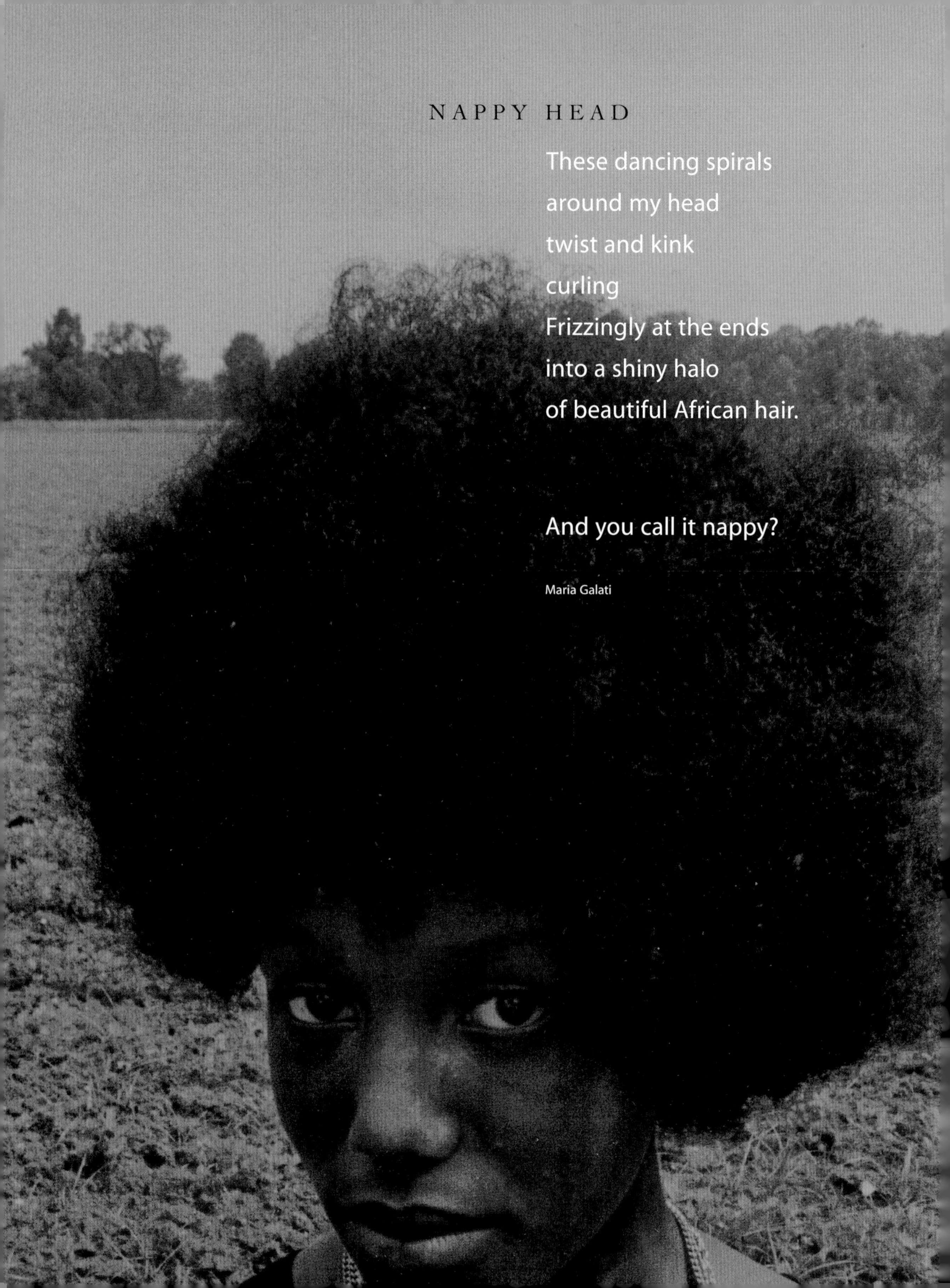

NAPPY HEAD

These dancing spirals
around my head
twist and kink
curling
Frizzingly at the ends
into a shiny halo
of beautiful African hair.

And you call it nappy?

Maria Galati

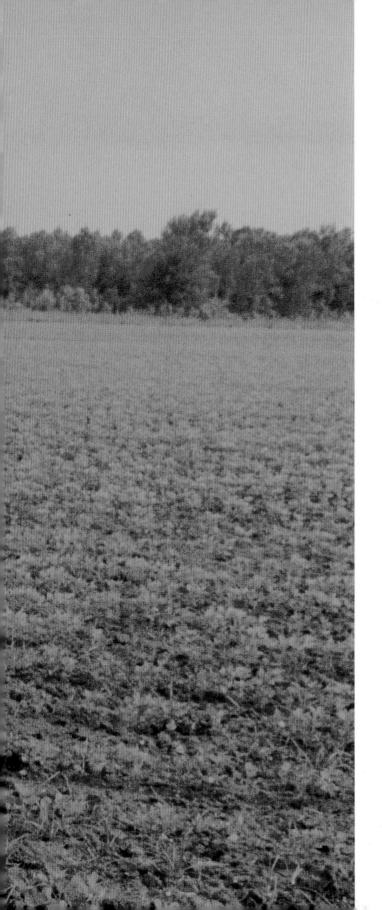

GOOD HAIR

dedicated to Roni Walter, founder of 'happi nappi wear' and Lonnice Brittenum Bonner, author of 'Good Hair: For Colored Girls Who've Considered Weaves When The Chemicals Became Too Ruff'

when I was a little girl
me and my friends had *good* hair
thick black
       happi to be nappi
greased, fried,
       lied to the side
rebellious, short, kinky and strong
twisted, braided, curly, snappy,
       wavy and long
we had good hair, cuz we had
black girl's hair

Stacey Lyn Evans

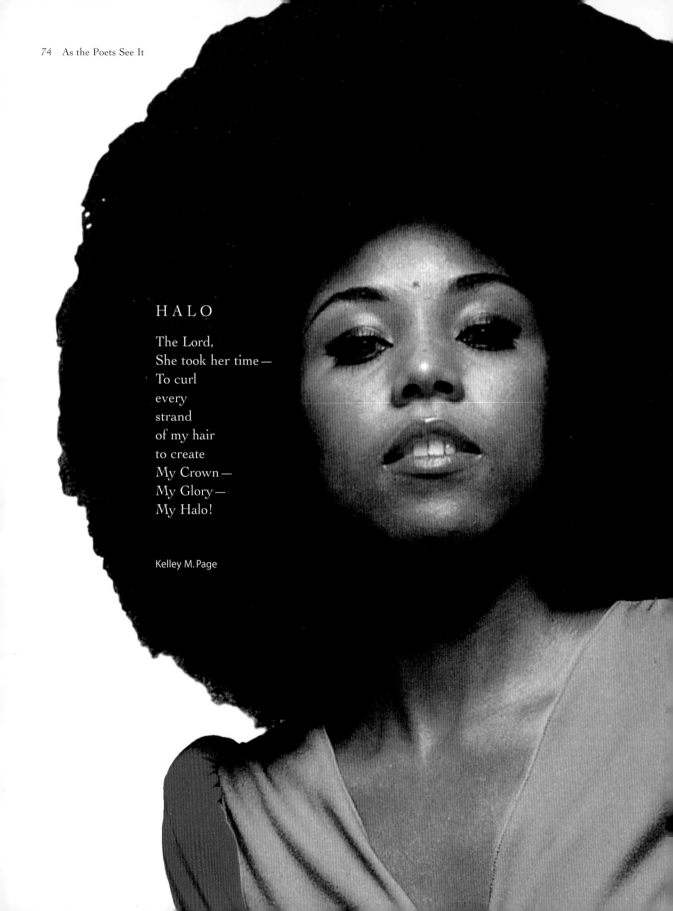

HALO

The Lord,
She took her time —
To curl
every
strand
of my hair
to create
My Crown —
My Glory —
My Halo!

Kelley M. Page

ON EXTENDING THE OLIVE BRANCH
TO MY OWN SELF

what was i doing anyway
was i crazy did i think
that by beating it into submission
i would win something
i've witnessed other casualties of war
the eyes of madness
that wandered through my neighborhood
after nam
what made me think
self-inflicted war would be
more merciful
or that oils & lubricants
metal combs of fire/chemical assault/all the
forces that modern technology could marshal
would ever win out over mother nature
& tell me this / what made me think
that would be a victory
anyway
a postscript
to my brothers and sisters:

it matters not how we wear it
but if we begin to wrap ourselves
just as tightly around each other & refuse to let go
if we rise up mighty like a dark cloud
& resist all efforts to change the nature
of who we really are
when we learn to stand
just as unshakable
in the beauty of our strength
and the strength of our beauty
then
then . . .

Harriet Jacobs

TO THOSE OF MY SISTERS WHO KEPT THEIR NATURALS

Never to look a hot comb in the teeth.

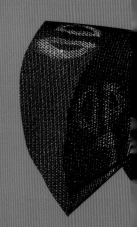

Sisters!
I love you.
Because I love you.
Because you are erect.
Because your are also bent.
In season, stern, kind.
Crisp, soft — in season.
And you withhold.
And you extend.
And you Step out.
And you go back.
And you extend again.
Your eyes, loud-soft, with crying and
with smiles,
are older than a million years.
And they are young.
You reach, in season.
You subside, in season.
And All
below the richrough righttime of your hair.

Gwendolyn Brooks

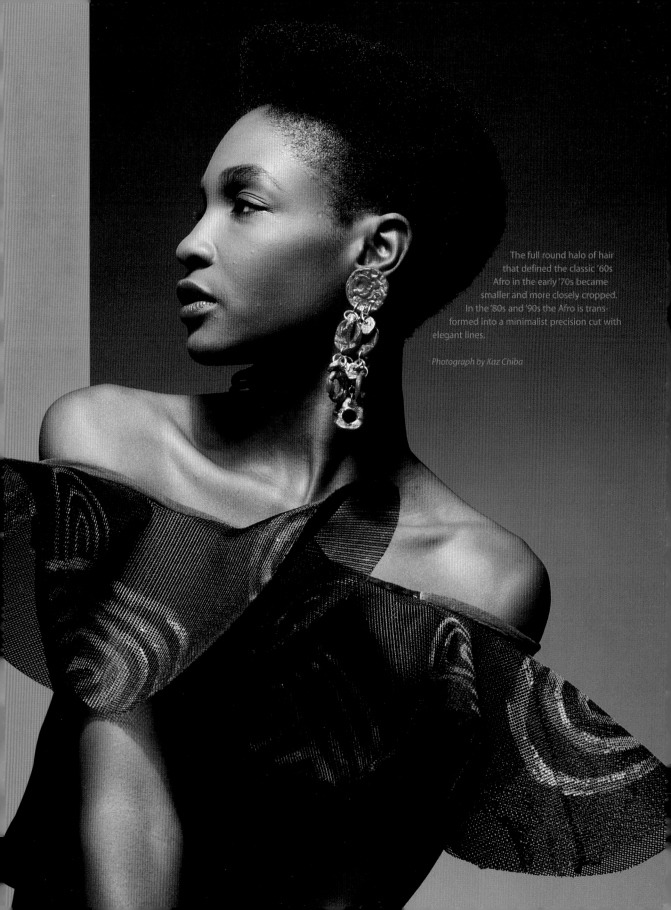

The full round halo of hair
that defined the classic '60s
Afro in the early '70s became
smaller and more closely cropped.
In the '80s and '90s the Afro is transformed into a minimalist precision cut with
elegant lines.

Photograph by Kaz Chiba

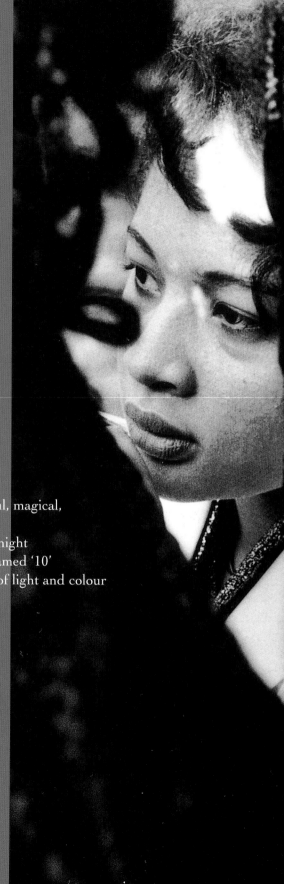

BORROWED BEAUTY

We've come full circle
from turban/headed women
(hiding cornrows)
in servitude;   cooking
              cooking
                 Suckling
              Cleaning
                 Cleaning
everlasting   Cleaning
              Cooking
                 Suckling

                 Cleaning
from turban-headed women
(hiding cornrows)
       to precious, time-driven 'dos
              to free-form Afros
          nocturnal braids escaping into
                       beautiful, magical,
       free-flying cloud Afros at
                    dawn, dusk, midnight
to our cornrows earning some woman named '10'
              magic money in flickers of light and colour
Do you know, Africa's child, woman,
black brown tan;
with our corn rows?
you are nobody's beauty but our own
and named   Sahara,
          Zaire,

              Cairo,
       Nefertiti
              Cleopatra
          Nigeria.

this is no borrowed beauty,
this is home.

Maxine Tynes

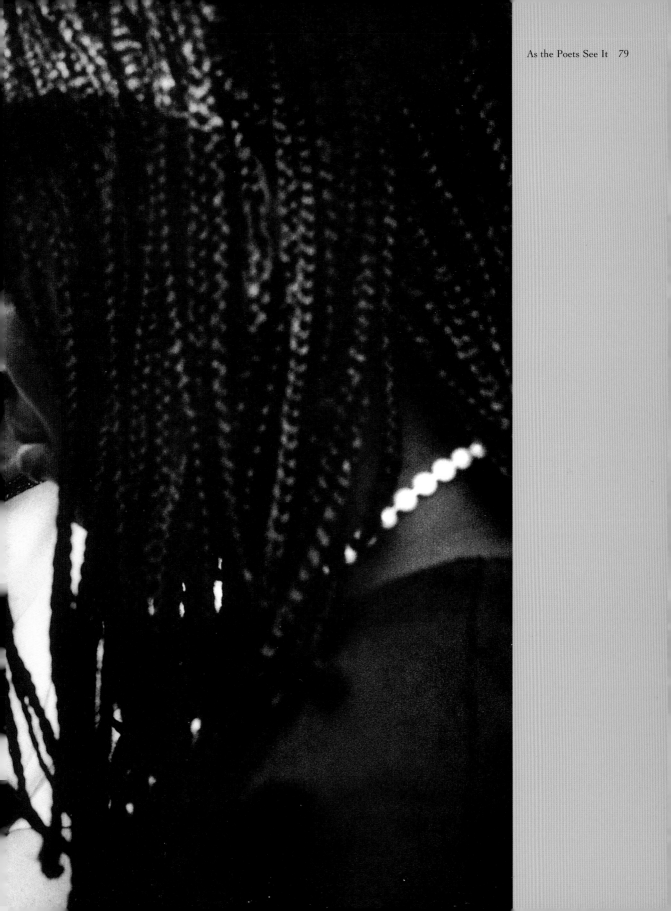

IF HAIR MAKES ME BLACK, I MUST BE PURPLE

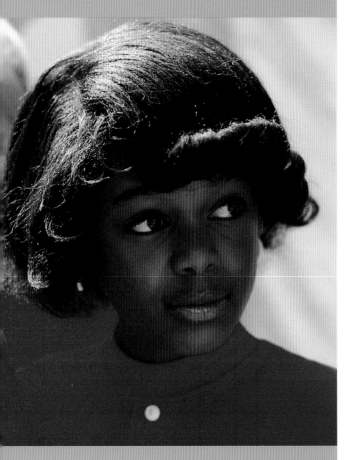

Yes, my hair is
Straight
But that don't mean that I ain't
Black
Nor proud
All it means is that my hair is
Straight

Because my hair is
Straight
Don't mean that I'm
Ashamed
And it don't mean that I want to be
White
Furthermore it don't mean that I ain't
Together

Yes, my hair is
Straight
And that don't mean a
Damned thing!
I am
Black
And proud
Knowing why

Linda Hardnett

GOOD HAIR

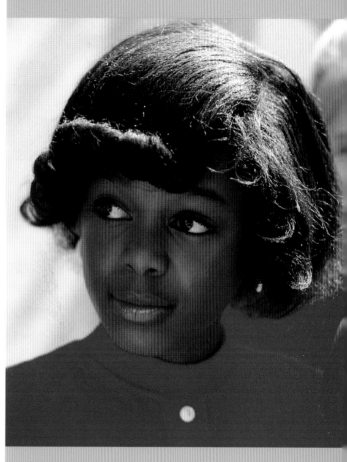

Early Sunday mornin' ritual
I can hear Moma's voice saying
Sit still girl
Bend your head
Unhunch them shouldres,
so I can get to this kitchen
Tight balled up hair
Don'tcha want it to flow like dem white
girls
My hair was stubborn
It fought a hard battle against
the straightening comb
Defeated it uncoiled
Fried into submission
Burnt ears, sore scalp
My cost for beauty
I look into the mirror at a strange image
Hair shiney, black and straight
I shake my head from side to side,
Like the girl in the Prell commercials
But my new hair laden with Dixie Peach
refuses to come out of place
Moma may not have known that I already
had a Royal Crown
But, Mother Nature did....
She sent the rains and my hair
went back home

Debraha Watson

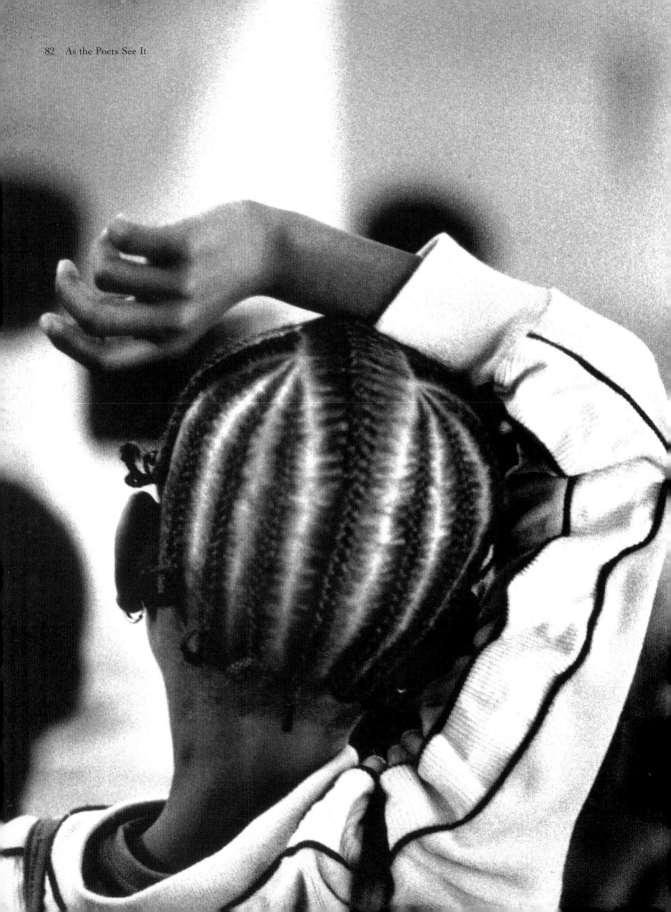

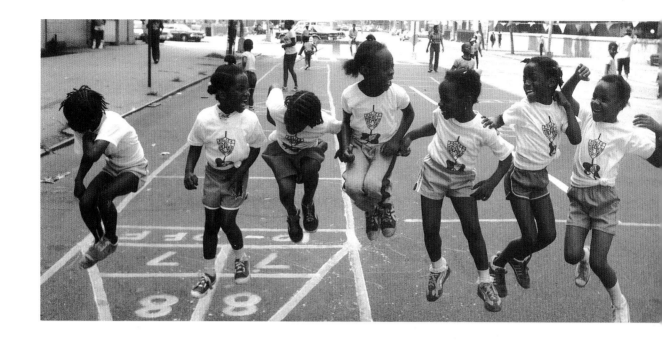

INITIATION

1.
Porch sitting hairbraiding
full of whys
questions for the faith
the rush of childtimes
slows the crafting of old hands
she wrangles my thickness into design
impatient arrows to the sun
fire from my head
the pull and rock of her ways
brings me back
done

she sends me out
the arrows reach
pull my back straight
i walk like a heron
clouds beneath my feet
looking into the sun
yellow becomes circles
circles bring out the creatures
zooming inside my eyes
the creatures make me dizzy
the sun puts me to sleep.

Monifa Atungaye Love

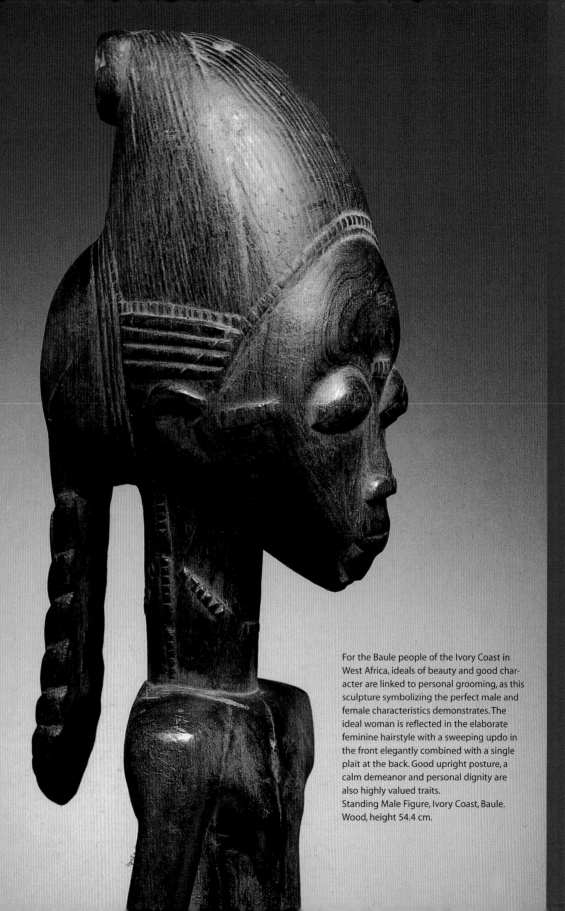

For the Baule people of the Ivory Coast in West Africa, ideals of beauty and good character are linked to personal grooming, as this sculpture symbolizing the perfect male and female characteristics demonstrates. The ideal woman is reflected in the elaborate feminine hairstyle with a sweeping updo in the front elegantly combined with a single plait at the back. Good upright posture, a calm demeanor and personal dignity are also highly valued traits.
Standing Male Figure, Ivory Coast, Baule. Wood, height 54.4 cm.

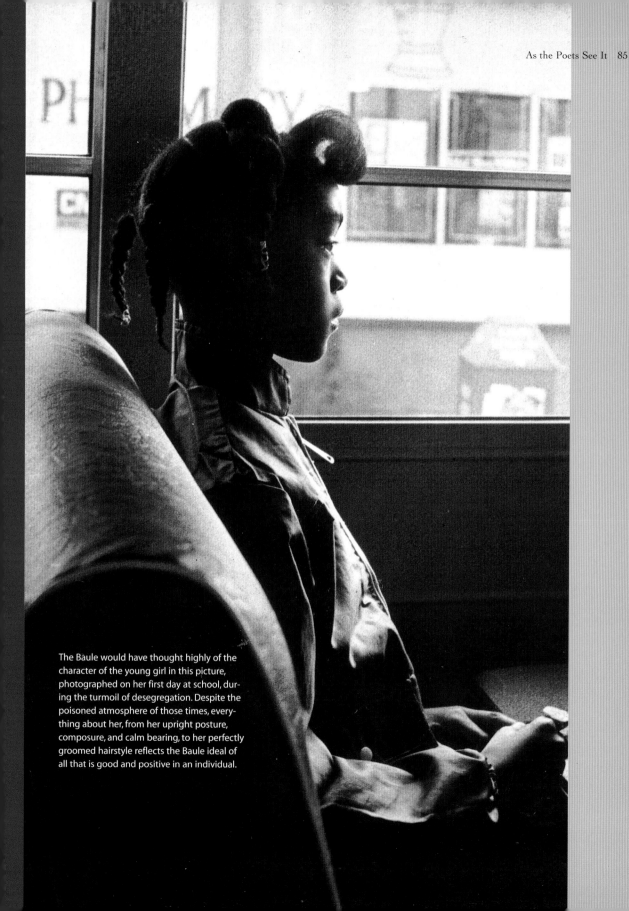

The Baule would have thought highly of the character of the young girl in this picture, photographed on her first day at school, during the turmoil of desegregation. Despite the poisoned atmosphere of those times, everything about her, from her upright posture, composure, and calm bearing, to her perfectly groomed hairstyle reflects the Baule ideal of all that is good and positive in an individual.

BY THE HAIR

People ask you:
—What did you do to your hair? —

You are colored
only non-colored people ask such questions
if you're colored you know
what coloreds do to their hair
in the beauty parlors
the unisex salons
the houses of style —
this is a custom particular to the colored.
If you're colored
the coloreds in the colored part of town know you
even if they don't know your name
they know your head
they know the colored you that's nigger and nappy
and kinky and wooly and dark
even when you no habla ingles
parce que tu parles français.
This habit you have of doing your hair
you learned it from your mother —
not that she thought being colored
was something less —
only, she thought knowing colored was not good enough
not straight enough
not manageable enough
not acceptable enough
to face a world that fears your difference
the darkness of you —
this is the custom of the country you live in
these are the ways of the colored in the country you live in
and people ask:
—What did you do to your hair? —

Why are scar tattoos on the cheek
marks of beauty
and the anorexic blond
the property of the white hunter?

Lois Griffith

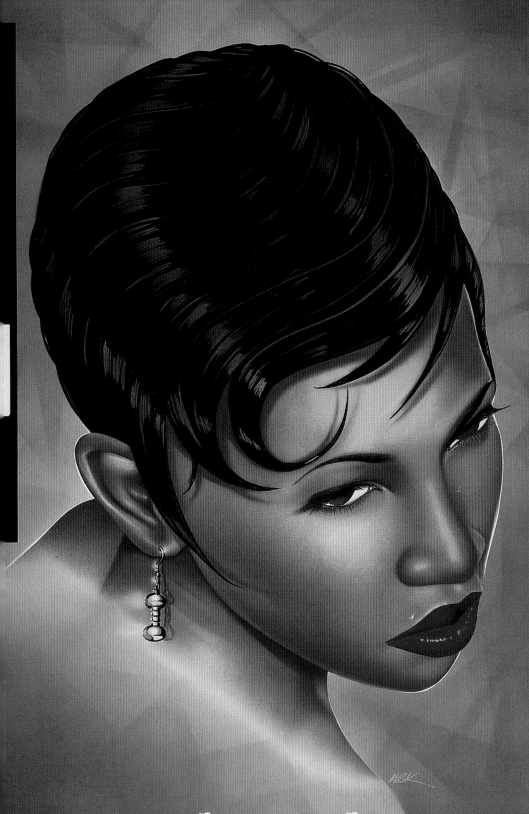

MULTiMOLD™

S, INC. 1000 E. 87th St., Chicago, IL 60619

HAIR WERKS™

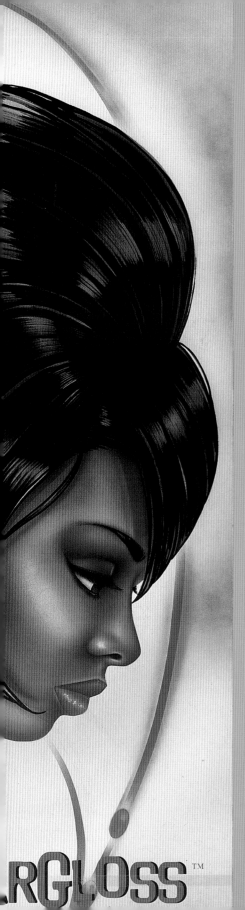

HAiR WERKS™

RGLOSS™

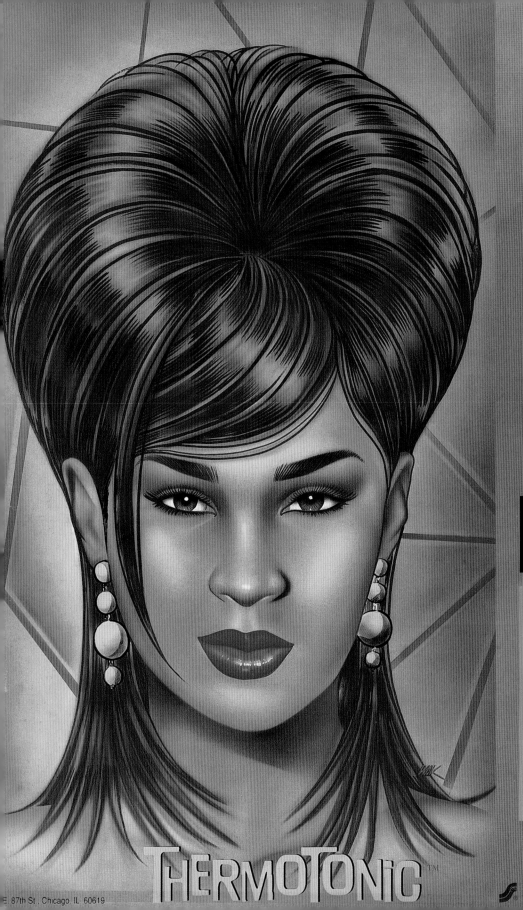

WERKS ™

HAIR ™

THERMOTONIC ™

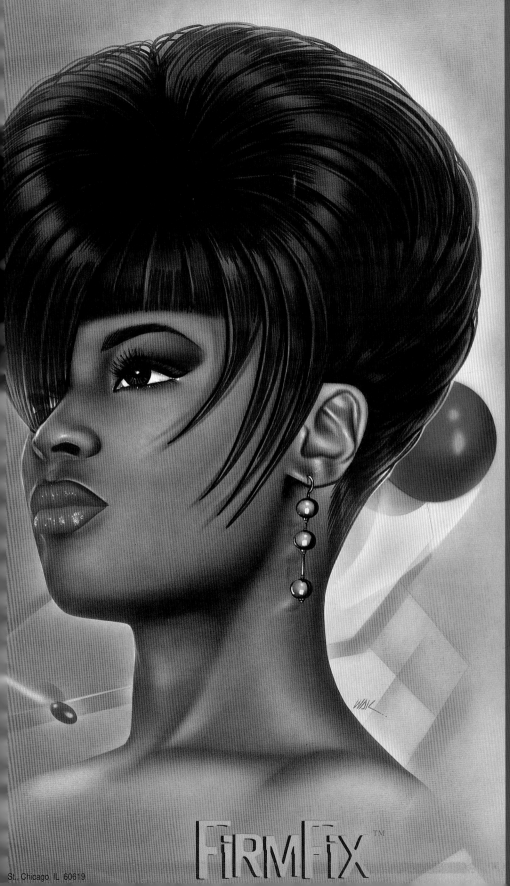

FirmFix™

St., Chicago, IL 60619

DREADLOCK

Saw you Dread.

On the first night
even though I perm my hair
& smoke way too much, in your absence,
jumped the broom with you anyway,
had two-point-five warrior-dreadlocked babies,
a dog named Mojo & a cat named Jubilee.

On the second night
saw you with a little white girl.
She was real small and pretty with dyed-
permed hair & a cigarette in her left hand.
You were earlobes & lips & syrupy sweetness

Saw you.
Dread.

Crystal Williams

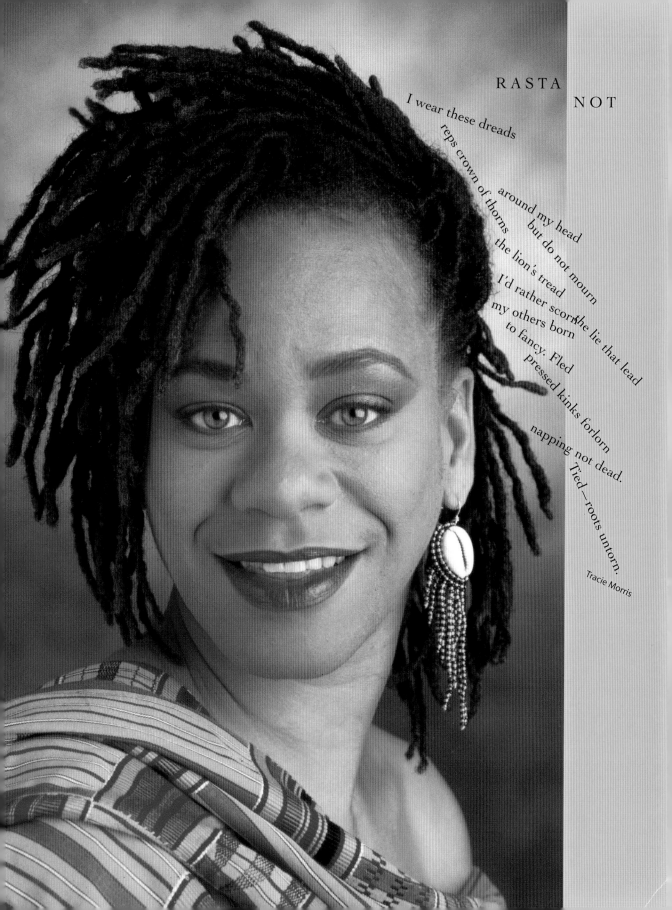

RASTA NOT

I wear these dreads
around my head
but do not mourn
reps crown of thorns
the lion's tread
the lie that lead
I'd rather scorn
my others born
to fancy. Fled
Pressed kinks forlorn
napping not dead.
Tied~roots untorn.

Tracie Morris

A HAIR POEM OF BLACK GIRLS

I.

How comely
this threshold,
the end of flesh

**like our blood
it presents,
a blooming.**

II.

Scrape to tips
hours singed,
pull away.

What gravity is
conveyed in
deep colors.

Those singed sunsets,
where round ears
mirror moons.

Tracie Morris

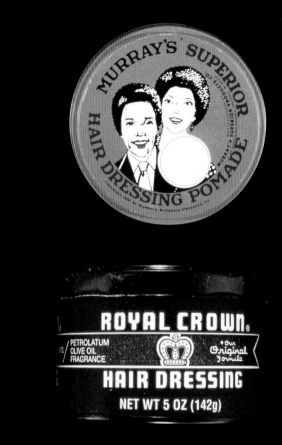

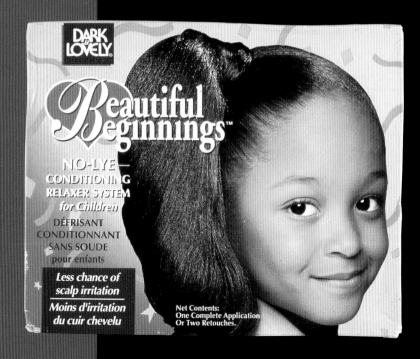

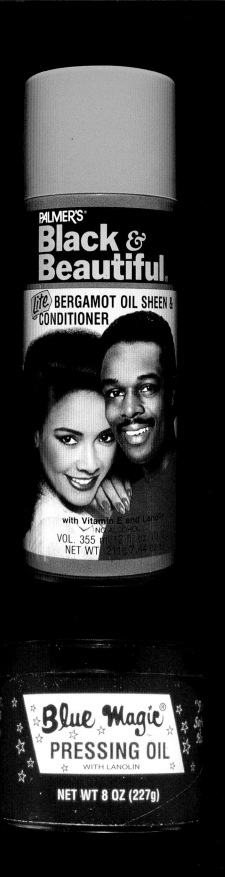

SOUTHEAST CORNER

The School of Beauty's a tavern now.
The Madam is underground.
Out at Lincoln, among the graves
Her own is early found.
Where the thickest, tallest monument
Cuts grandly into the air
The Madam lies, contentedly.
Her fortune, too, lies there,
Converted into cool hard steel
And right red velvet lining;
While over her tan impassivity
Shot silk is shining.

Gwendolyn Brooks

ROOTS

I am sorry you are
proud of the man
who raped your
great-great-great
grandmother and left
your hair good.
Please, this is not
envy it is sorrow
for the long road
we must travel
to be sisters.

My lineage
can be traced
through the roots
of my hair to
Nairobi.

Do not
try to make me
ashamed Of this
fact, sorry my hair
grows in dry tight
cottonfields on my
head and will not
fly in the wind
like the woman I am not.

Charlotte Watson Sherman

European artists who accompanied explorers on expeditions to the continent often made sketches of African hairstyles. While their colleagues occupied themselves with finding minerals and crops to exploit, these artist-travelers keenly observed and recorded local customs and traditions. The drawings and sketches from the earliest expeditions from the sixteenth century onwards provide documentation of the rich creative legacy and social history of African hairstyles. Melton Prior, Special Artist with a nineteenth-century British expeditionary force clearly recognized the rich variety of hairstyles of Ghanaian women. In a feature story in the *Illustrated London News* of April 4, 1874, he published his sketches of "Female Fashions at Cape Coast Castle," what is today the West African nation of Ghana. Melton Prior noted:

> "The headdress is a gay kerchief, with sometimes a bunch of feathers, grass, or flowers, put over the women's hair, which is twisted into a variety of shapes, knobs, ridges, and tails, as shown in our illustration; the figure at the upper left hand corner of the engraving shows the rough hair before this artistic process."

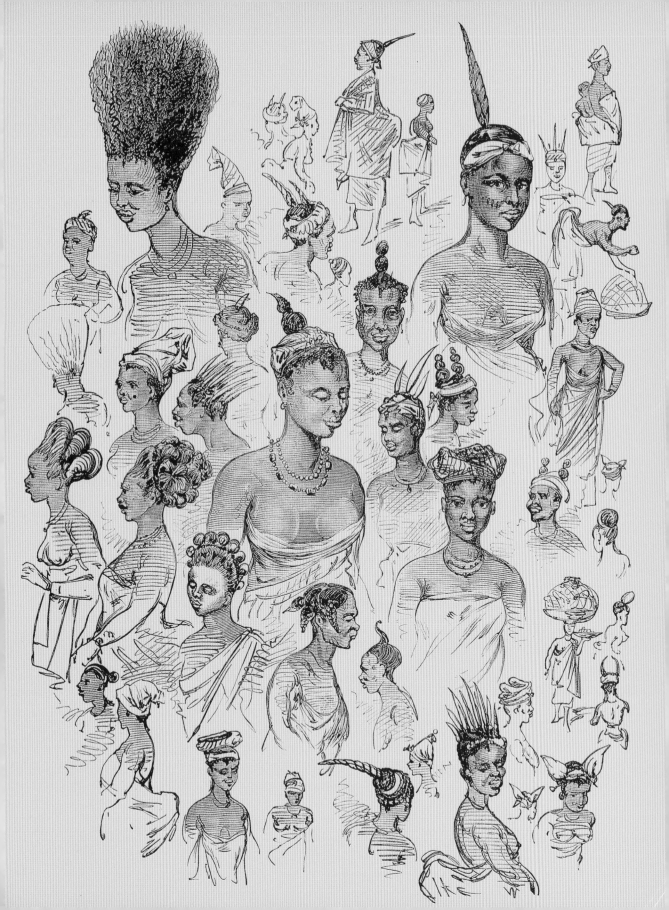

MY FIRST LOVE

My first love be
Hair
natural
ain't washed for weeks
Hair
the myrrh and the musk of it
Hair
the lilac blossomin'
of ancient shrubbery
Hair

parted by rivers
of grease and kink
Hair
a plantation of jujubes
cultivated by tender hands
Hair
agitated to tremblin' bliss
Hair
unruly comb-breakin'
Hair

burstin' hematite and obsidian aglow
Hair
eternal smokin' afro bush
with a black power fist
raised like a pyramid
Hair
outta control forest fire
approachin'
your city
Hair
that drifts
and grows
shamelessly
in touch with the deep-grown roots
of the fertile land
called scalp
Hair
she be my first love.

Jennifer McLune

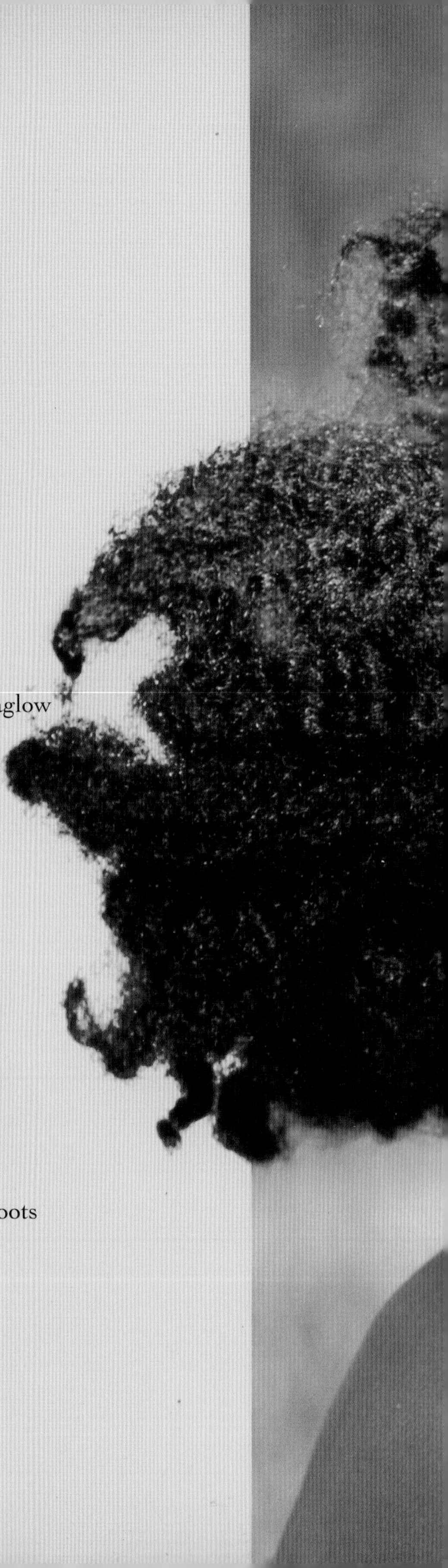

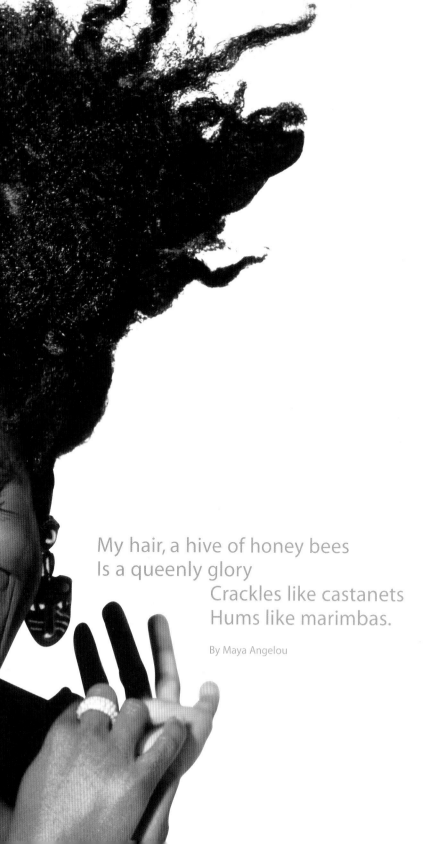

My hair, a hive of honey bees
Is a queenly glory
Crackles like castanets
Hums like marimbas.

By Maya Angelou

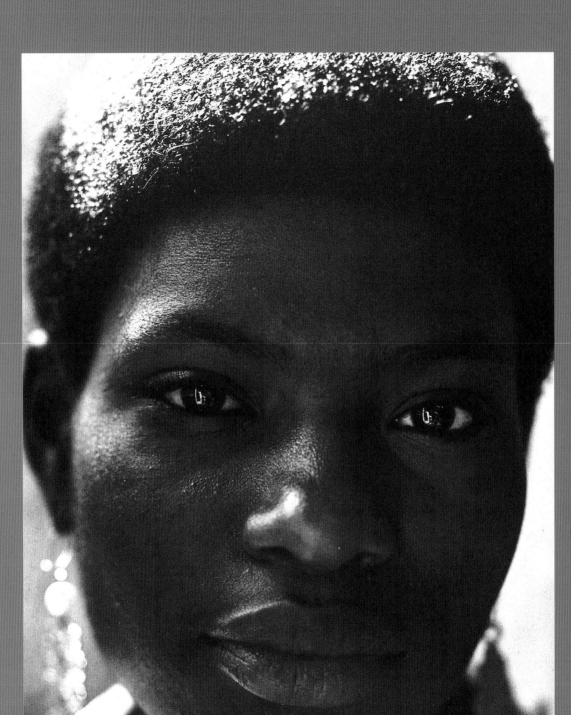

THERE'S HISTORY IN MY HAIR

I once read a poem
about the politics of hair
then afterwards looked in the mirror
and wondered when I was little
in my coal colored halo of kink and frizzle
did a prevailing stick straight world
see a nappy, ugly me

I mean could they see all the way to Africa in my eyes
my nakedness, my culture exposed enough for them
to wish they had a missionary at hand
to civilize, sanctify me
a little girl who proudly wielded a pink ace comb
and volunteered at school
to comb their naturally silky hair

I was young
called it playing beauty shop
only realizing years later
even then, how beautiful I was
with my tawny skin unlike crushed pearls
my mahogany eyes more deep, sparkling
than those blue as cerulean skies
where across flew the bird of privilege, paradise

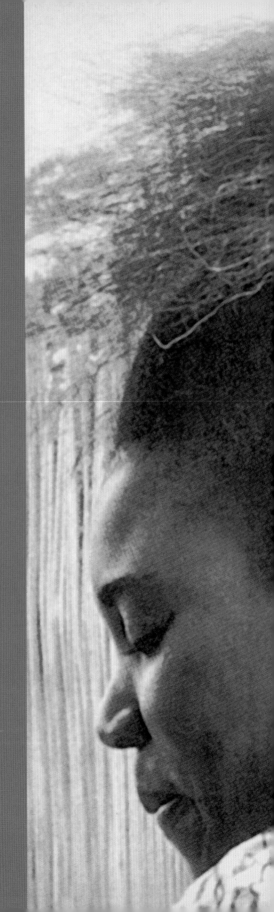

I was young, then
a fledgling phoenix still waiting to
be born
and to think all this came
from reading a poem
from examining the politics
of my skin and hair
and realizing
even as a happy, nappy little girl
how phenomenal
how compelling
how infinite
my beauty was
and still is

Karen Williams

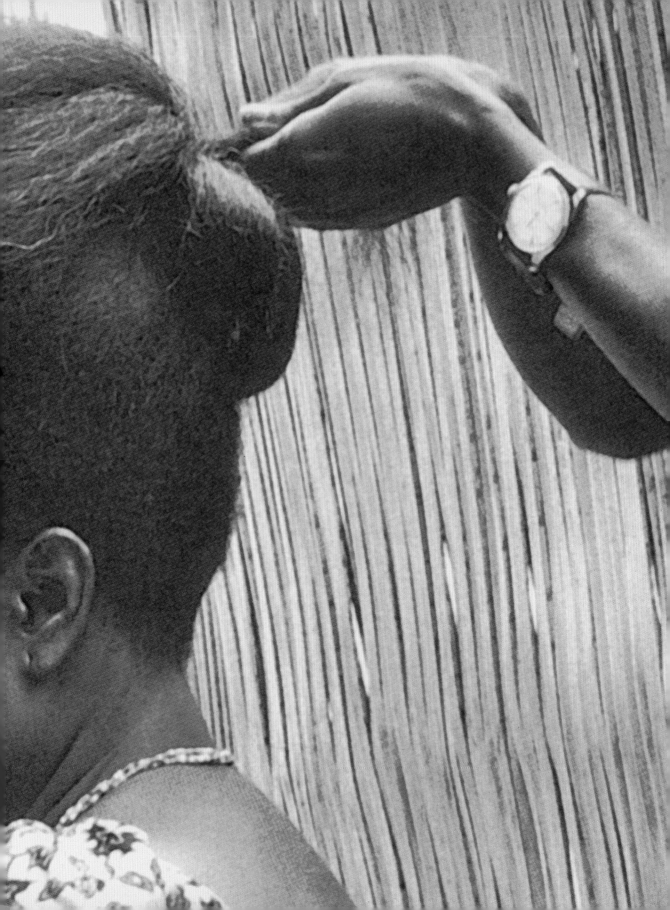

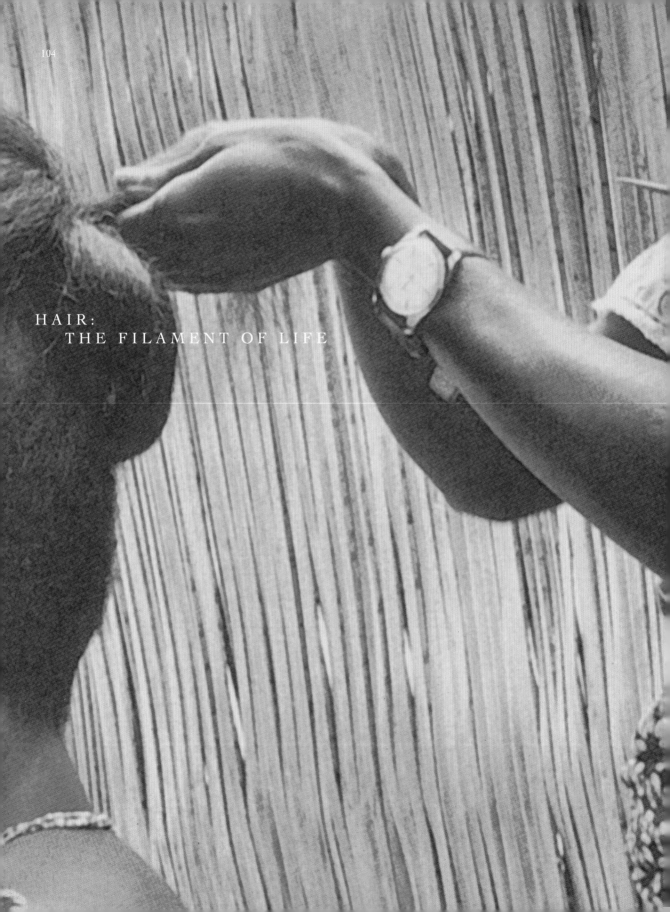

HAIR:
THE FILAMENT OF LIFE

Hair they say it still grows after we're dead
just like memories antique curios we keep in silver boxes
and by then in the casket
it's not good hair or bad hair
or nigger hair or white folk stringy hair
it's just hair
gray slivers of moonlight
a ripple of raw gold
deep as an otter's skin caked with mud from a long forgotten sea
a molecular tapestry of cuticle cortex root still oddly alive
key to a private dark world more vital than its keeper
filled with carnivorous worms
bits of decomposed flowers
a still shining wedding ring

When living we lose over 50 to 100 strands of hair per day
in the normal combing brushing and fussing of hair
When living it lures is a sexual symbol
says if worn loose and free
we too are loose and free
ready to take on man
to be whole in a man's world
When living we use it as a battle ground
Mama says keep it. We say cut it

The print-dressed woman with wild children 'round the way
says to my coal-colored halo of kink and frizzle
Lawd! Dat chile sho' got bad hair
while to me it's just hair
black beautiful just like my mother's and father's
my grandmother's still growing in the grave
the hair of Isis once a charm to breathe life into Osiris her dead lover
hair she spread over her children the wings of an eagle to protect them from harm
strands of dead cells
Delilah's Circe
A gift of the Magi deeply rooted to life.

Karen Williams

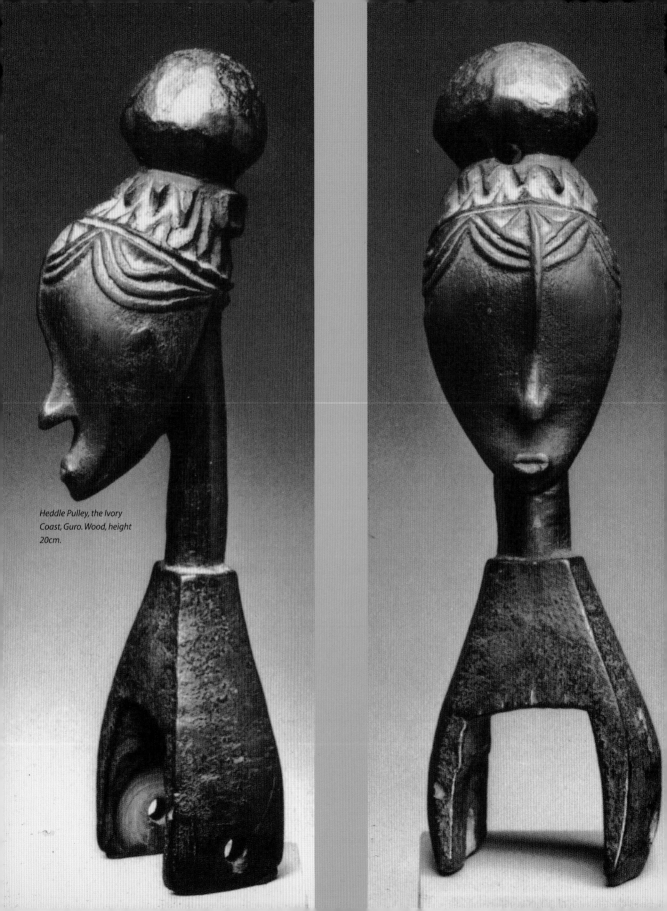

Heddle Pulley, the Ivory Coast, Guro. Wood, height 20cm.

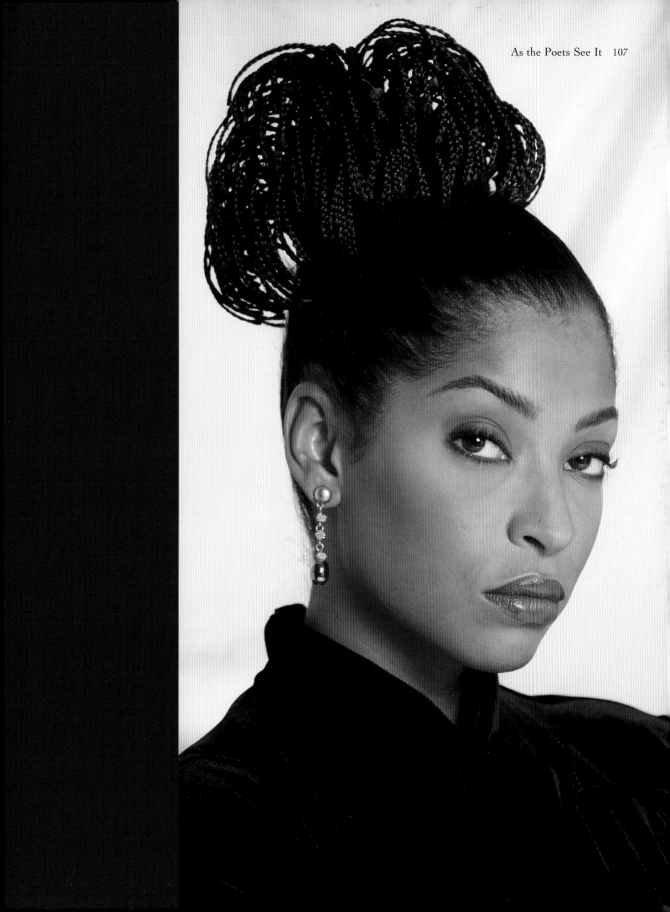

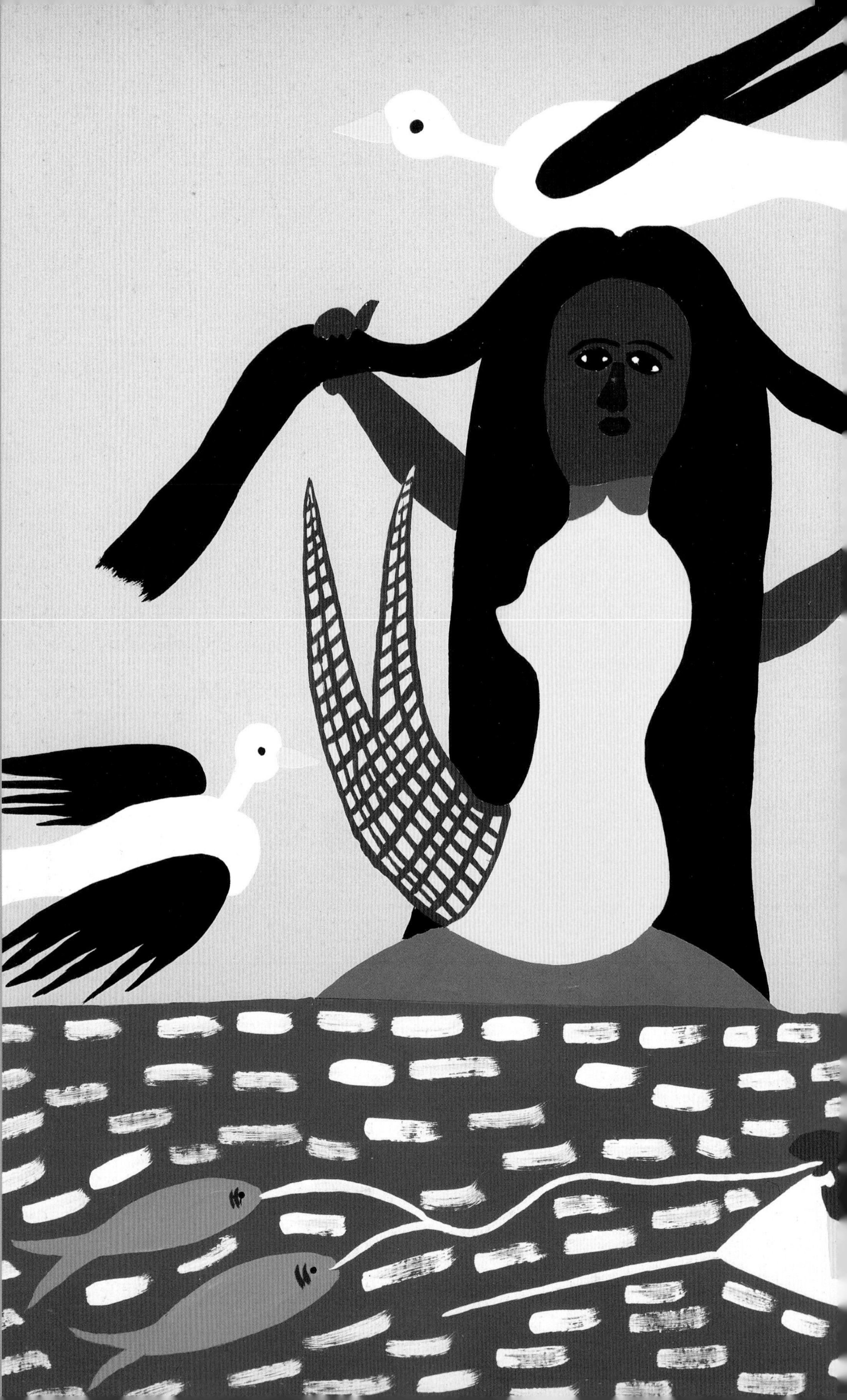

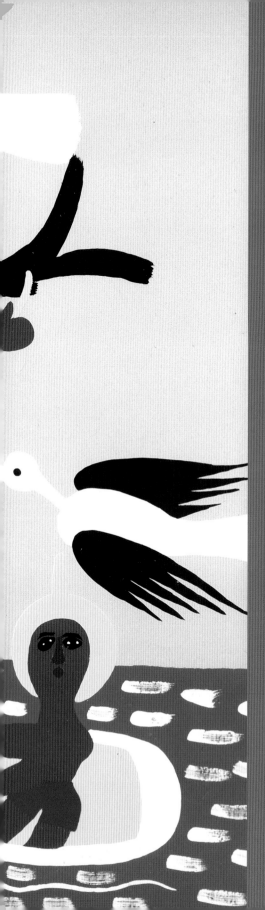

MERMAID

Legends and myths about mermaids and the sea are
present in virtually every culture of the world, and this
is also the case in many parts of sub-Saharan Africa
and indeed throughout the African Diaspora where the
legend of mermaid known as Mami Wata still thrives.
In parts of west and central Africa where the network
of rivers are linked to the livelihood of the population
the legend of Mami Wata is particularly strong. She is
the guardian of the sea, bringing good luck, health and
riches to those who honor her, but she can be equally
dangerous, causing victims to drown or boats to cap-
size if not properly respected. To placate this capricious
siren, paintings of the mermaid appear in sculptures,
wall paintings, and on family altars and appear as
good-luck charms on all sorts of objects, from key rings
to jewelry to T-shirts. Long hair is an essential part of
Mami Wata images as Amos Ferguson's painting
shows. In most African countries long hair is especially
prized, not as we often think of it as part of the good
hair/bad hair debate, but because long hair that is thick
and strong is associated with health, vitality, and
fecund qualities.

Scenes from the Salon

ANNU PRESTONIA,   SALON OWNER

In 1989 or 1990, I had been doing hair for about two years and every-body used to say go to *Essence,* but I was reluctant, I had known people who had gone up there and had gotten their work rejected, so I felt it was not time. A friend of mine wrote an article about African hairstyles and submitted it to them and along with pictures of my work. At that time many women in the mainstream, especially those not involved in African culture had not seen such a wide variety of braids. When the saw the article, I had women calling me from places that I did not even know black women inhabited, like North and South Dakota, Europe, Canada, and Alaska. The article caused a really big explosion This was an idea whose time had come. The phone calls to the salon went from five or six a day to seventy.

On Hairstyle Names

I give names to my styles since we have to describe what they are. I just come up with catchy names. The problem is that because this is a relatively new industry, so everyone comes up with different names and it can get confusing.'

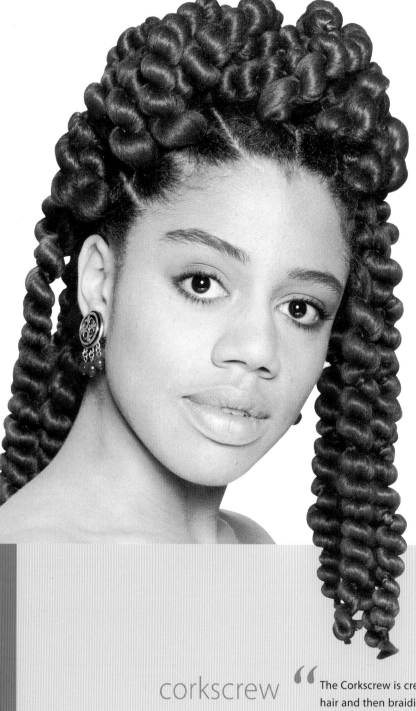

corkscrew " The Corkscrew is created by sectioning hair and then braiding it with a long thread called weaving or button and carpet thread. Leslie started coming to me when she was about fourteen years old. She has the most incredible amount of hair I've ever worked with, its extremely thick, it used to kill me. This particular style did not take as long as most, it only took about four hours."

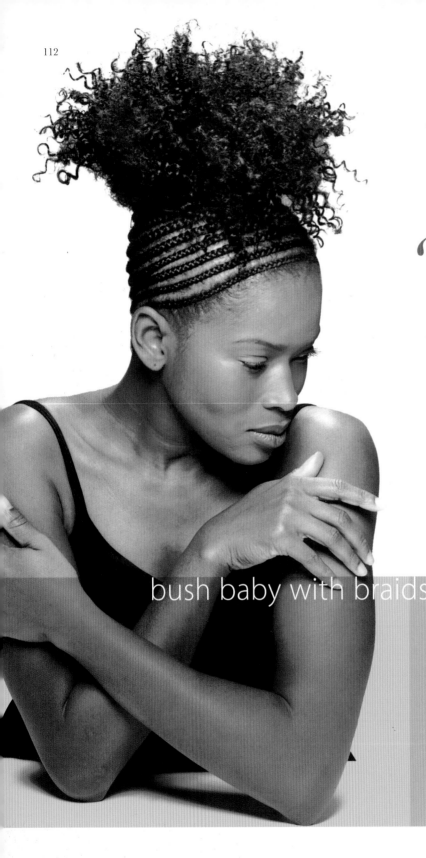

bush baby with braids

"This version of Bush Baby is done with braids, so it's more versatile because it's not a weave. You start by braiding the hair from the root, and then you weave the extensions into the braided hair, leaving them partially undone so that it's full and loose, which gives you the style. This is a really popular style. I think the popularity of styles has to do with things that are happening socially, the images that are seen in music videos and are promoted as sexy. I think to have a lot of hair has always been promoted as sexy. There used to be a time when you could not have this texture hair unless you were born with it. For a long time people wanted straight hair, but increasingly the mulatto look, where the texture of the extensions is a mixture of Caucasian and African, became popular. To get the hair extensions this texture, it is chemically processed. They wrap it on rods to get the curl pattern and then appiy the chemicals on it while it's on the rod, which holds that texture."

"Goddess braids really took the popularity of braiding to a new level. When they came out they were so different because everyone at that time was trying to get braids small, and the smaller they are the more technique required, which takes more time and skill and therefore more money. All of a sudden here were big braids that could look beautiful. Up until then, most big braids had been ugly. This style came out of Florida, and it was just so elegant that I coined it Goddess braids. With this style all those closet people who wanted braids but thought they would never, wear braids came and asked for these styles. A lot of them were hair-dressers who worked with straightened hair and only wore curls. When we did the hair shows, a lot of hairstylists would line up and ask for this style because it was a look that allowed them to retain their hair texture and still look good with braids. This style took ony two hours at the most."

goddess braids

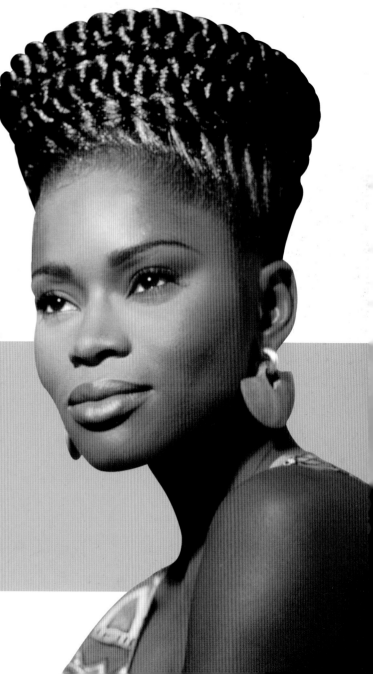

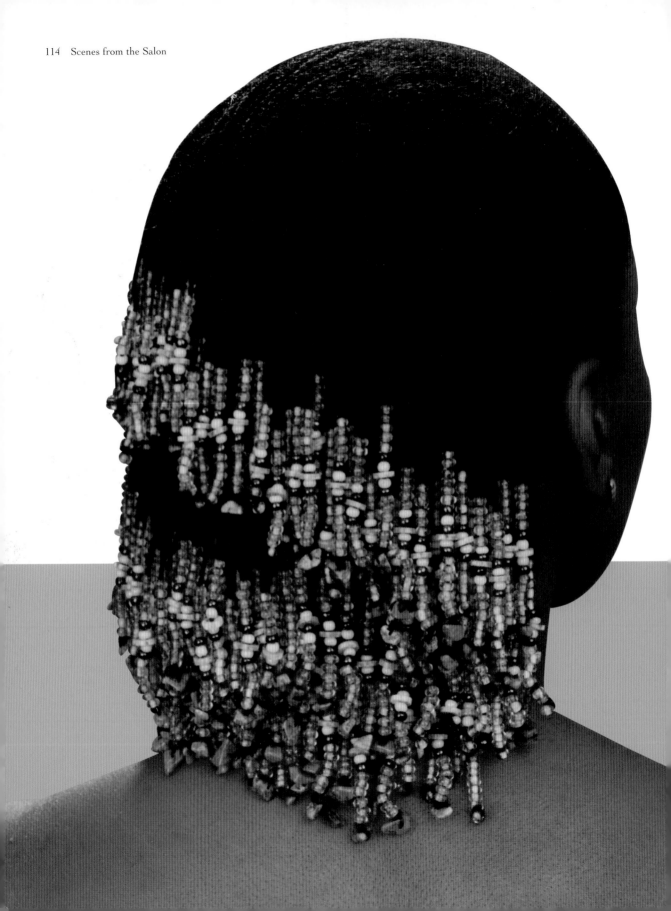

beads

"The beads started the whole braiding [interest] for me, that's when I started doing braids. I was living in Washington, D.C., and I went to a family picnic and heard this woman say that she had seen a friend of hers who had her hair braided and paid twenty-five dollars. I thought to myself, how ridiculous, I knew how to braid hair, and thought I would NEVER pay anyone to do my hair, it was just unheard of back in 1977. Then I saw someone with a wonderful hairstyle and thought it was something I had to get done. By then, the price of braiding had gone up to sixty dollars, I paid it a couple of times, even though I was a student at Howard and could not afford it. So I started doing my own braids, and the next thing I knew I had clients. The best part for me is shopping for the beads and putting the colors together, I love colors and trying out different combinations. The braids have to be extremely small in order to get the beads thread through each braid. This was definitely a two-day hairstyle. Working in a twelve-hour stretch, the model had to come back the following day for a period of six hours. First you braid the hair, and then you string the beads through each braid, and then the ends are tied to stop the beads from falling off."

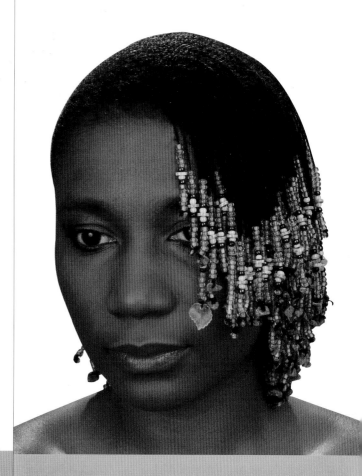

starter locks

the cherokee

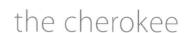

" I love this style, it makes anybody who gets it look about ten years younger. I had it, and I loved it, it's very flattering on almost anyone. It's basically a large size cornrow that's done very long to give a Native American look."

" Starter locks are ever so popular, this is a style that is used to start the process of locks. When you first get locks you are basically training your hair to grow in a new way. Once your start the locks, you have to come in every four to six weeks to get it shampooed. When this happens the lock pattern basically gets washed out and you have to curl the shape again. It's a bit like getting a set, you apply setting gel to each lock, and you roll the curl shape on a comb. The wash and re-curl process is repeated for about five times, until about the fifth time the curl begins to remember the lock pattern and starts to grow in that way."

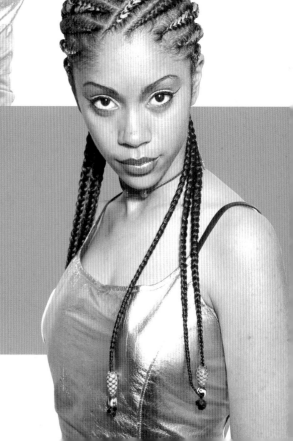

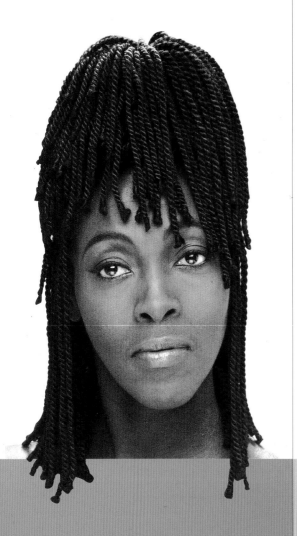

senegalese twist

" When this style came out it was very big. the first time I saw it was on this woman. It was gorgeous and had to ask 'where did you get your hair done?' I would have gone anywhere to have it, and I ended up going just where she said which was Senegal. I could not find out how to do it so I ended up going all the way to Senegal to learn the style and especially to get the fibre. The style is done with a special cotton candy-like fibre called Laine. I brought some back with me and had it a year, and despite my visit I still could not figure out how to do the style. Finally I met this woman from Senegal who showed me how to do create it. When this style came out around 1987, we were basically producing it everyday at the salon. Just about every client was get-ting the Senegalese.Twist.Then the source of fibre dried up, it was hard to get the Laine in America. I once waited three and a half months to get my hair done because I would only have this style and nobody had any Laine in New York. This model was a very special friend of mine, she persuaded me to branch out and hire more satff, she had a warm personality. She was a very special person. We just started out our woman's organization in memory of her."

"These cornrows were braided by starting at the hairline and going back toward the middle of the head. Each braid consists of three individual pieces of hair that are crossed one over the other in alternating motions which gives you a braid that fits flat on the head. These cornrows were done with extensions making it extremely elaborate. It took about eight hours."

cornrows

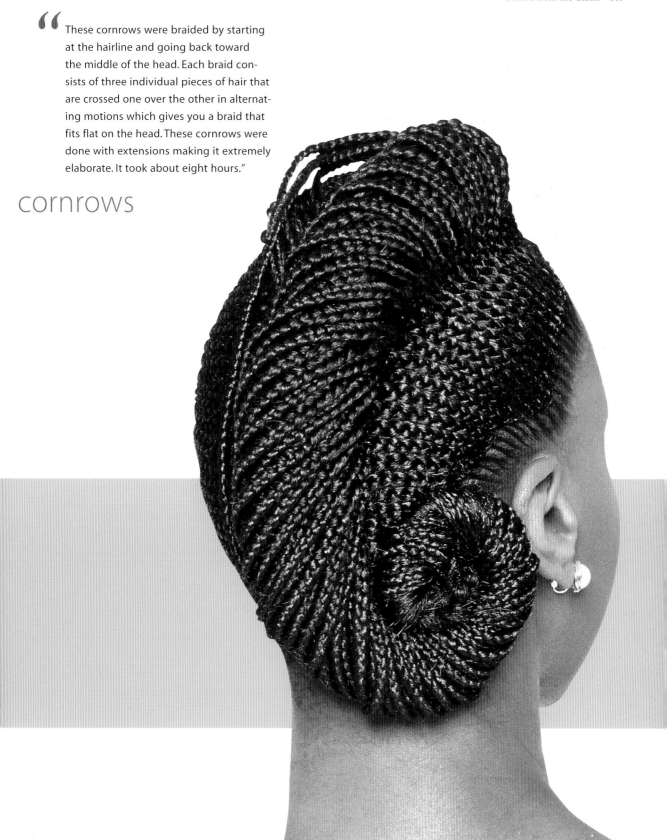

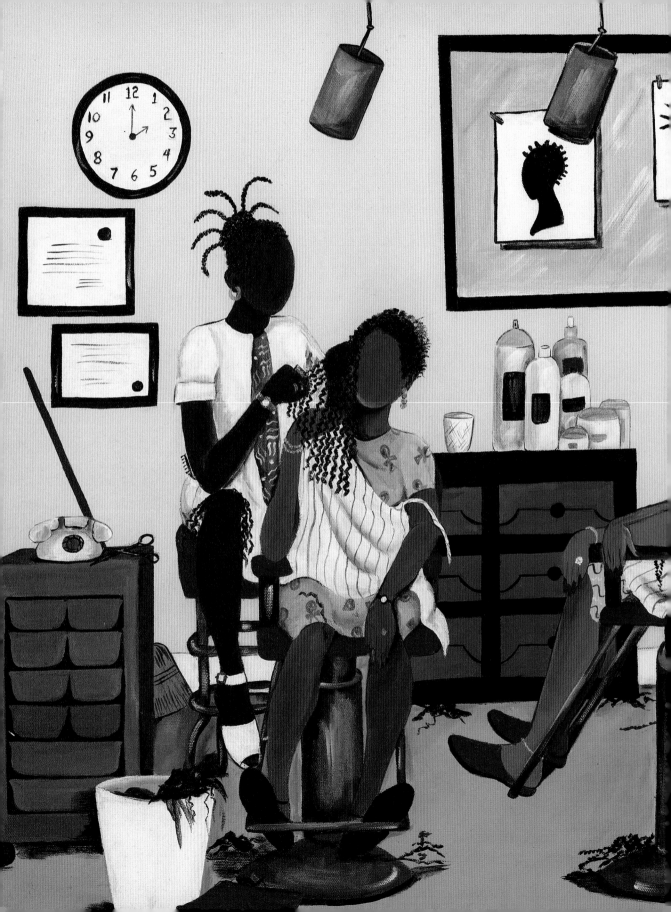

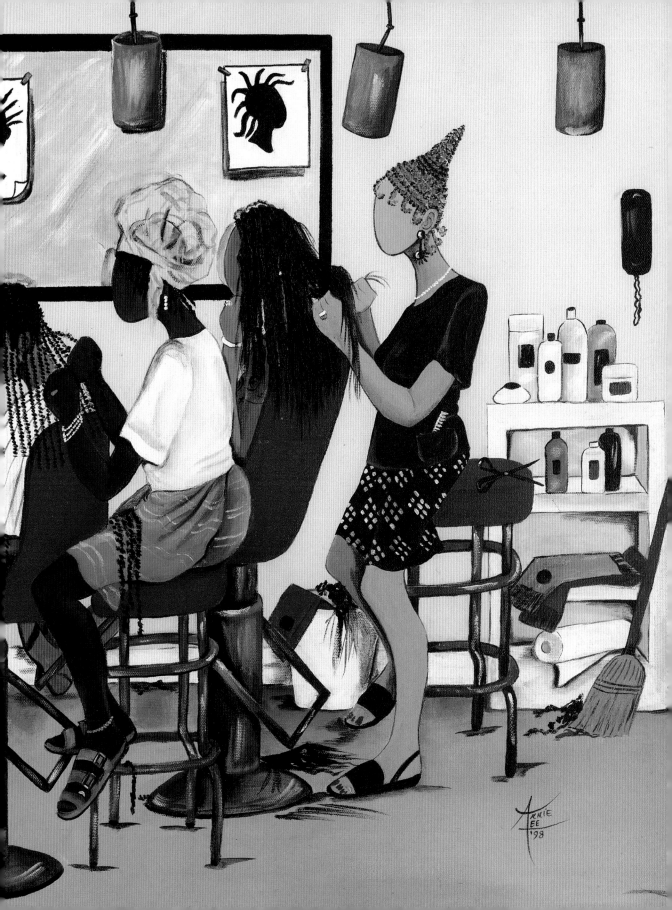

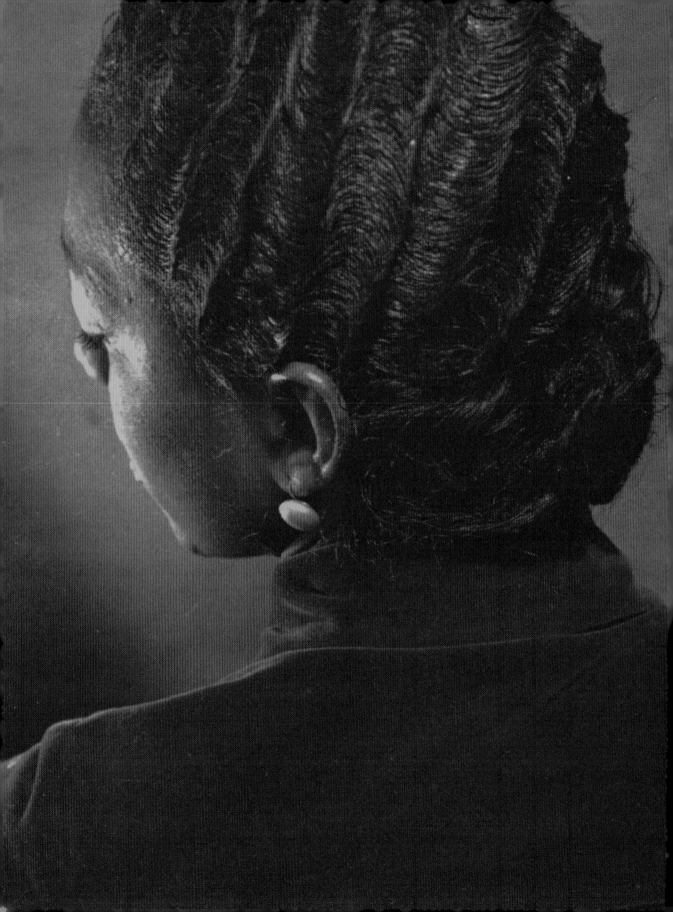

The finger wave hair style was very popular in the 1920s and 30s. Hairstylists of the time turned it into a high art form in which the amount of curls and the pattern was only limited by the skill of the hairdresser. The look could be seen on women everywhere, especially in the society columns of the *Amsterdam News*, back then Harlem's top newspaper. Finger waves were also featured in advertisements, beauty school instruction manuals, and graduation portraits of the 1920s and '30s. The finger wave craze ended by 1940, and it was not until the late '80s to early '90s that the style came back more popular than ever. It was even the topic of a lawsuit. Like all hair trends however, it went out of vogue by the mid-90s.

Seven Steps for Stylish Finger Waves

1. Wash and rinse hair.

2. While it is wet apply generous amounts of gel or, preferably, *Creamy Set.*

3. Comb hair straight down in the direction you want the curls to form.

4. Starting from the top of the scalp down to the back, use your finger to make a wave by pushing the index finger forward until a small ridge pattern is formed.

5. Continue to make the wave impressions all the way back to the back of the head.

6. When you have finished making the pattern,sit under the dryer until hair is dry and wave pattern is set.

7. Apply hairspray to give hair sheen.

STYLIST NOTE
Creamy Set is a setting lotion brand preferred by many hair professionals because it dries without leaving small dandruff like flakes that some hair gels leave. Finger waves look best on short to shoulder length hair. Your style should last two to three days, after which you will no doubt notice it begins to look tired.

Style information courtesy of Margaret Hitchcock of Ebony 2000 Salon.

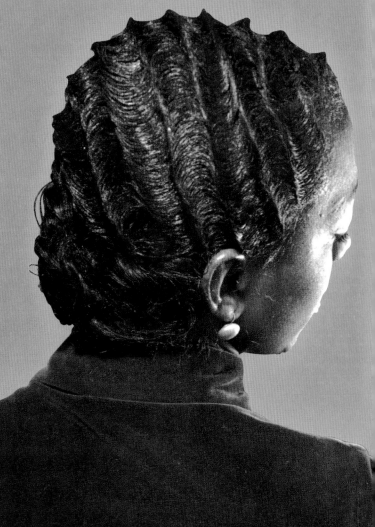

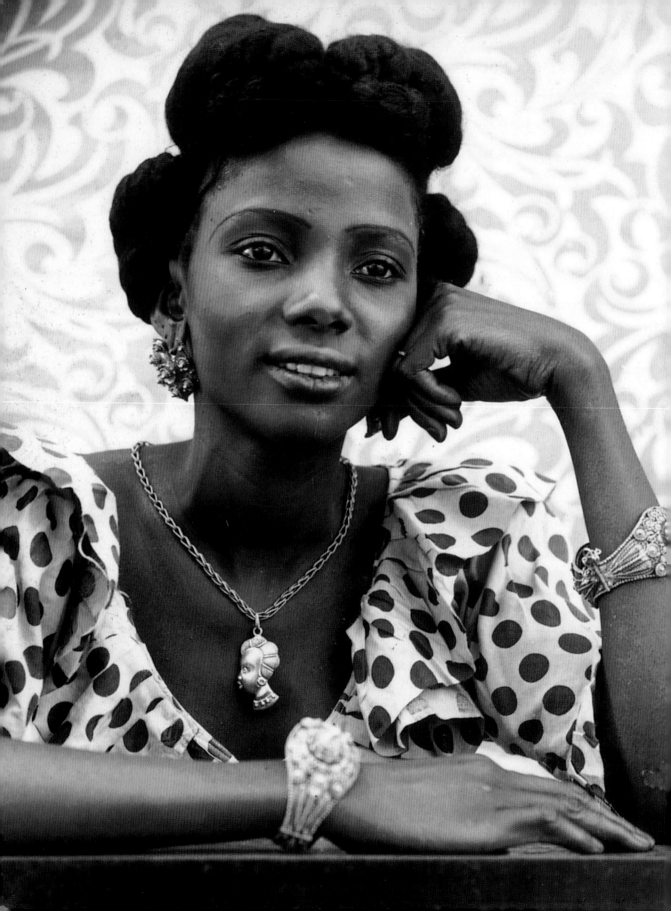

A Wolof woman from Senegal, West Africa with hair curled and tied with wool. She is wearing earrings and bracelets decorated with "buttons" (Kulalaati) and a silver pendant with the head of a Fula woman from the region of Guinea whose hair is braided in a popular helmet style shape.

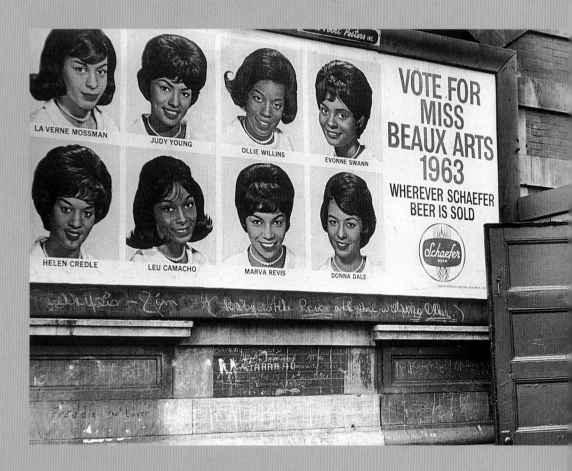

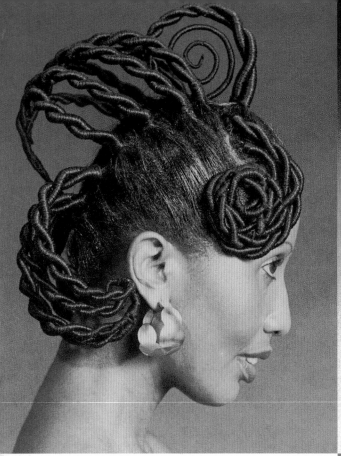

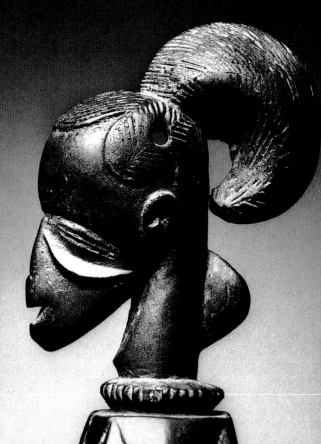

This elaborate hairstyle was achieved by wrapping black thread around strands of hair, a technique called thread plaiting or thread braiding. It is particularly popular in West Africa and especially among Yoruba women.

This wood sculpture made by a Guro artist from the Ivory Coast in West Africa, provides us with clues as to what traditional African hairstyles looked like. The elaborate curved piece at the back could very likely have been created by cornrow braiding, or more likely by thread plaiting, a popular technique in West Africa, in which black thread is wrapped around strands of hair. Thread-wrapped hair, which feels like wire and is just as flexible; strands can be tied together or bent into shapes only limited by a braider's skill and imagination.

Heddle Pulley, Ivory Coast, Guro. Wood, height 16.5cm.

This hairstyle is typical of young Shawan girls in Ethiopia. The front of the hair is braided in small cornrows and left loose at the back. Hair is kept shiny and conditioned with rancid butter, a popular form of moisturizer in this region of Ethiopia.

This equally flattering African-American equivalent of the Shawan hairstyle reflects the historical links and shared culture of the black Diaspora. By the 1960s, opportunities for travel greatly increased the two-way traffic between Africans and African-Americans contributing to the free flow of old and New World culture. Rap, hip-hop, permanents, Soft-Sheen, L'Oreal and other brand names have become a part of modern life in Africa, while in America, cornrow braids and other traditional African hairstyles continue to grow in popularity.

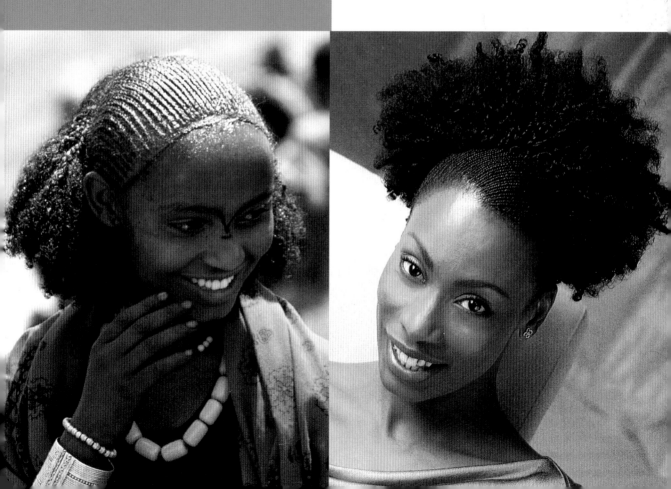

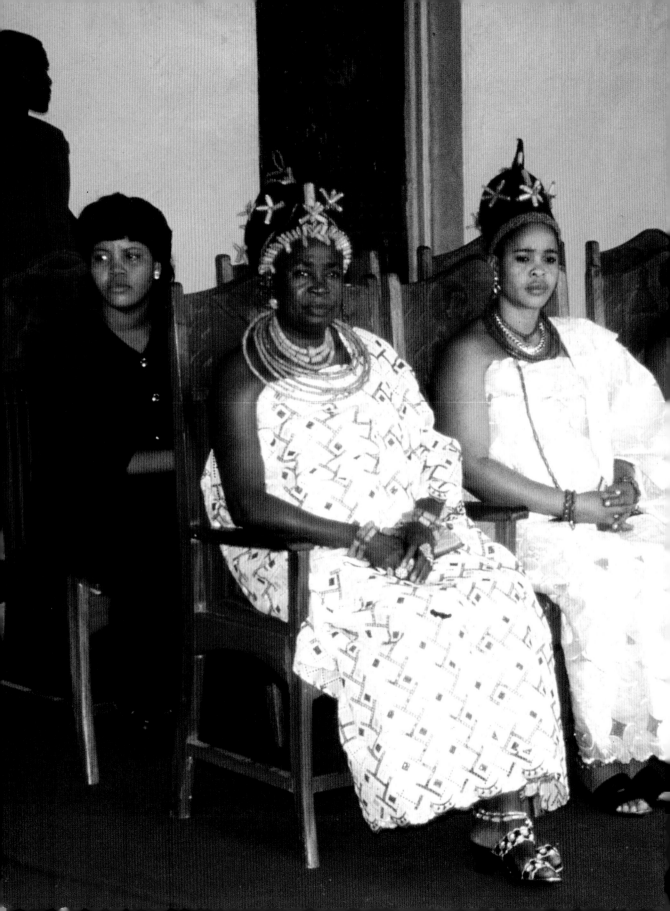

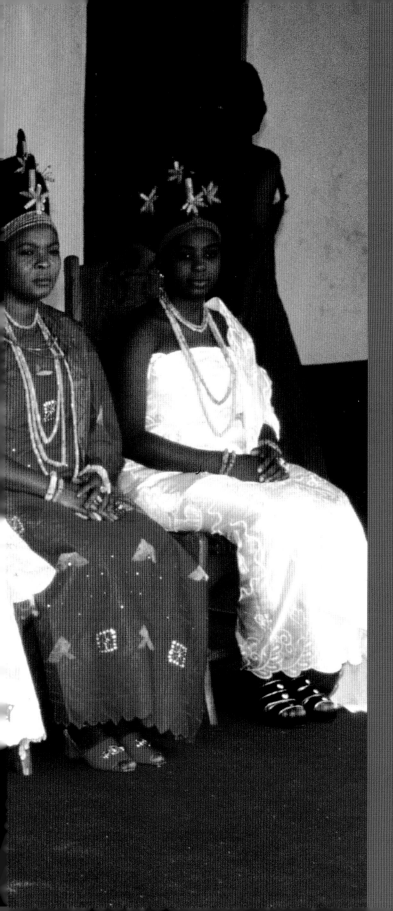

CHICKEN'S BEAK

In most African countries, traditional hairstyles are still worn today especially on ceremonial occasions and other significant events such as weddings and funerals. Hairstyles often have particular meanings and often define a woman's status in society, such as marriage or a special social role. Here, women of the royal household of the ancient West African Kingdom of Benin, in Nigeria, wear an elegant and elaborate hairstyle called "chicken's beak." The "chicken's beak" style, which dates to the eighteenth century, is created by carefully brushing and building up the hair to give a beehive effect, the hair is then decorated with gold and coral trinkets. The rank and seniority of each of the women is defined by the amount of coral jewelry used, as well as the size and styling of the pointed peaks.

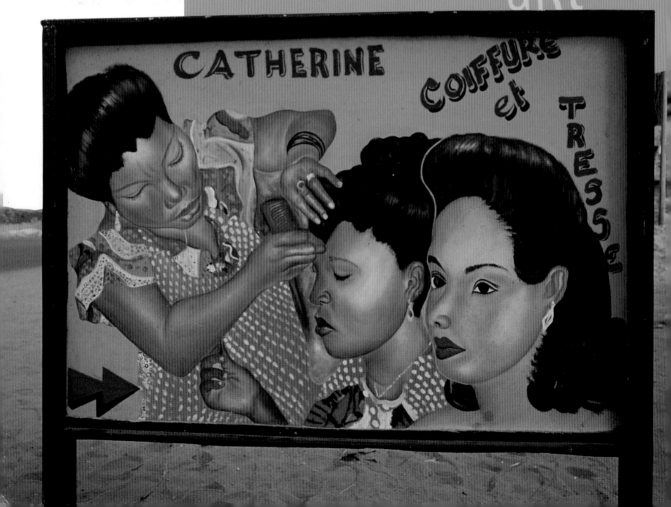

ADVERTISING ART
ADORNS AFRICAN CITIES

From Abidjan in the Ivory Coast to Libreville in Gabon via Kumasi to Ghana and on to Lagos in Nigeria, Africa's city walls and shops play host to a vibrant display of popular art.

This colorful form of advertising emerged over the past forty years as urban populations swelled along with economic development. These hand-painted artworks sing the praises of local small businesses. The vivid images illustrate the commerce that hums from sun up to sunset along streets, in open markets, and in improvised wooden storefronts. The artists paint on *banco* (sun-hardened clay bricks) or cement depending on locally available supplies and the financial means of the trades people.

Advertisements for hairdressers and barbers are leading examples of this art form. The paintings announce the presence of the hairdresser in even the smallest corner boutique, but more important, they inform passersby of the latest fashion and the newest products.

Painted in minute detail, the artworks show women just how their new hairstyles will look. Creating these expensive hairdos for customers attending parties or family ceremonies takes the hairdresser many hours of painstaking work. The beauty salon itself is a meeting place where chatter and gossip fill the air, punctuated by joyful laughter.

These elaborate hairstyles started out as a form of ethnic and sociological recognition. Today they are a way to develop and display a prestigious form of individual style. Women's magazines published in the Ivory Coast and Nigeria have popularized the styles throughout Africa.

The painters and the hairdressing advertisements first appeared in the 1950s. These ads were probably the first works by these primitive artists drawn by the powerful charms of the cities to leave their villages.

Back then they were all self-taught relying solely on their own invention and imagination. Today, most of the sign painters are specialists. Their livelihood is tied to the small businesses that bring the economy to life, publicizing their services by decorating their shops and signs.

One of these artists, Bitok T. Pierre, has painted exclusively beauty parlor signs since 1964. Thanks to the quality of his art, this painter from Cameroon has been the favorite of the Libreville's hairdressers since 1969. He works in close collaboration with his clients. They choose subjects for him to paint from fashion magazines and hair-care product packaging. His style has continuously evolved, always changing but always maintaining his initial sense of joy intact. Today he's reached an artistic pinnacle with the results on view in an open-air gallery for all to enjoy. To see the show, a visitor needs only to head for the center of one of the city's poorer neighborhoods, for it is here that the creative beat of these artists and their patrons throb. Together they have invented a symbol of the artistic vitality of the common man, an ode to the joy of life under even the most difficult circumstances.

Jean-Marie Lerat

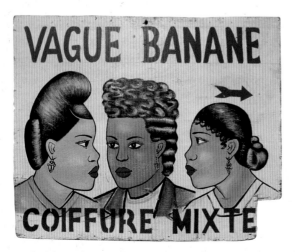
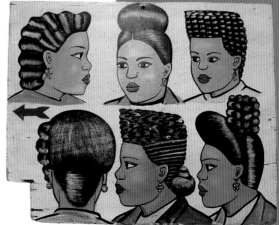

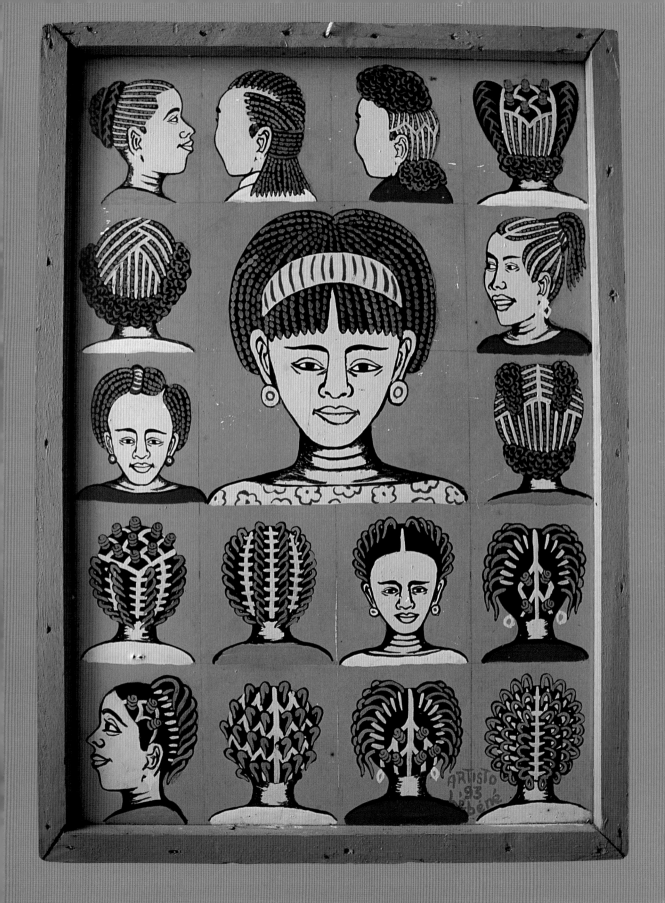

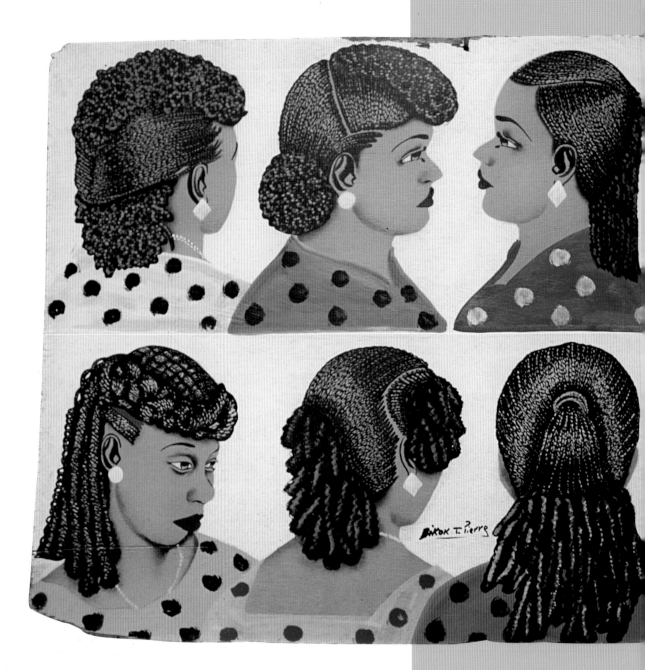

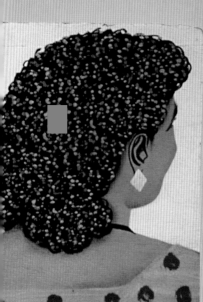

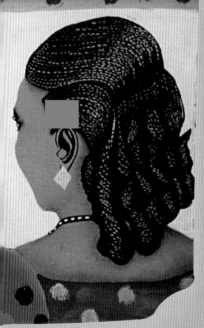

Hair braiding from the simplest to the most complex styles are created all over the African continent, and although styles vary from region to region, braiding goes back centuries, and is an age-old art, steeped in rich social traditions and customs. There are hairstyles for married women, for young girls, styles for ceremonial and religious occasions. Some styles are dated to the nineteenth century and resemble traditional African sculpture from nineteenth century as well as drawings made by nineteenth-century travelers and explorers.

Nina Gwatkin

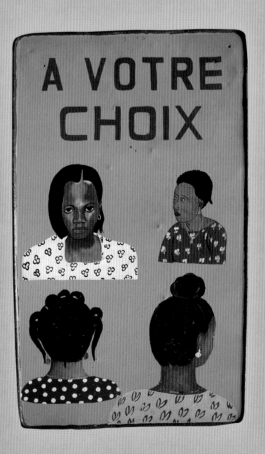

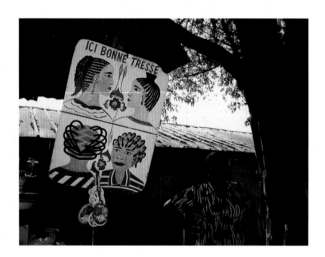

THE ART OF HAIR BRAIDING

To begin the hairdressing, the hair must be clean and fully dry. It is first combed out into a "bush" before being roughly divided into sections. Pomade is applied, and the hairdresser then begins the meticulous parting that will bring out the final pattern. The hairdresser skillfully varies the chosen style according to the shape of her customer's head and the length and thickness of the hair. Once the hair has been straightened, it cannot be arranged in any plaited styles because it does not have enough body. The completed hairdo will usually last about a week before a return visit to the hairdresser is necessary.

Braided hair can be made into long fat twists or short small braids that stand out from the head or can be worked into thin plaits (cornrows), which lie close to scalp. Cornrow style braids are created by taking thin parallel sections of hair, which are then parted off. The hairdresser then takes up a very few strands at the beginning of a section and works them into a threefold braid. More hair is worked into the braid as she proceeds along the row until there is a thin braid all along the middle of the section; she repeats this process for each section. The braids may begin from the crown of the head or from anywhere along the hairline, and each variation has a different name.

Nina Gwatkin

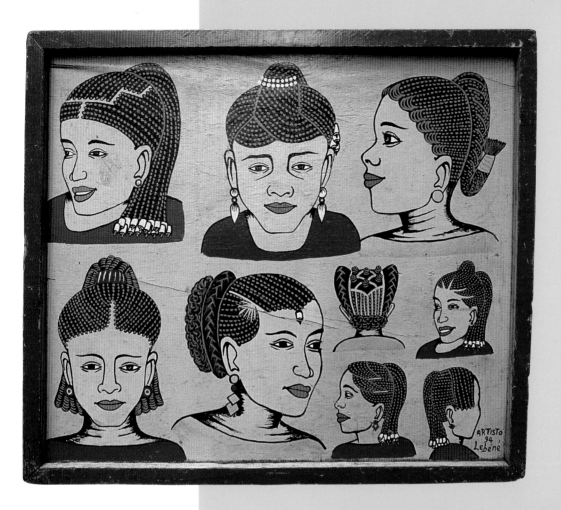

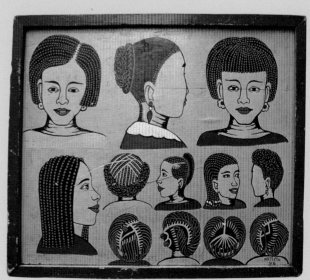

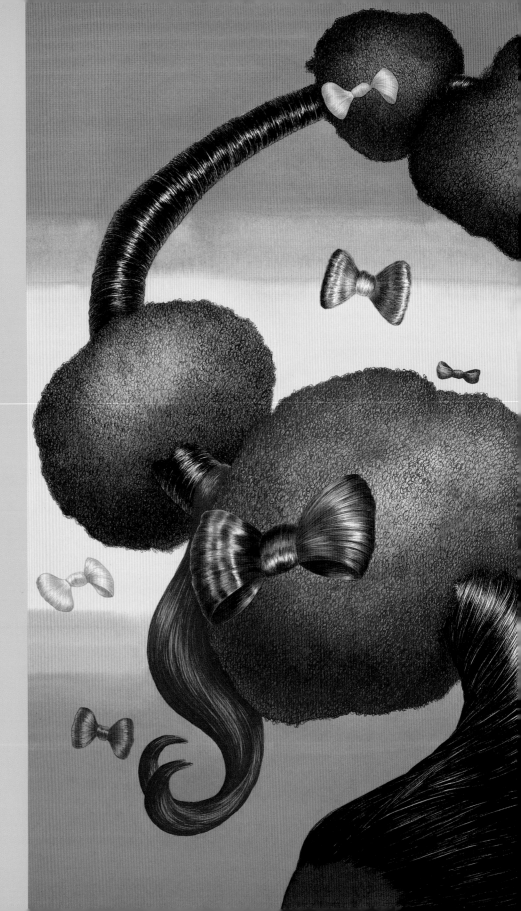

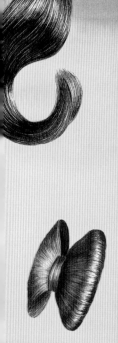

"Black women may not be natural blondes, but they do know how to mix blondness with hip-hop attitude and blues-singer soul."

Veronica Chambers

color
color
color

TeCHNicoLor hAir

color

BLOND LIKE ME

Beautiful blonds, from Marilyn to Madonna, have come in all
shapes and sizes. But African-Americans with blond hair are a new
twist. What began as merely outlandish—a platinum-tressed
RuPaul, a yellow-haired Dennis Rodman—has hit the black mainstream. Years ago, the black poet and activist Audre Lorde asked
her Afro-wearing sisters, "Is you hair still political?" The answer
then was a strident yes. The answer today is less prone to rhetoric.
Yes, no, sometimes.

Jada Pinkett, the actress, sports a satin-blond marcelle that makes
her look a lot like the model Naja, except shapelier and with a better tan. Nikki Giovanni, who was once called "the princess of black
poetry," has also gone stark raving blond, proving that the revolu-
tion will not only be televised but colorized as well. Homegirls like
the rapper Pepa of Salt-N-Pepa buy their blond hair by the yard,
weaving it into stylish shoulder-length braids. As a host on the Sci-
Fi Channel, the futuristic songstress Grace Jones wore a plasticized
bright yellow wig.

Purists see blond sisters as traitors to the race. At Town Hall
recently, black intellectuals gathered to watch a discussion between
the Harvard professors Cornel West and Henry Louis Gates. Some
poor woman with blond dreadlocks was almost booed out of the
room as she walked to her seat. "Who does she think she is?" was a
common refrain. "Deranged," hissed the woman beside me. Well
known as a race man, the director Spike Lee has been doing a lot of
explaining for his wife Tonya's natural blond hair. In an *Ebony* magazine interview, he pleaded: "Please tell people that my wife doesn't
bleach her hair…. It's her natural color."

Mary J. Blige, the singer, is undeniably black, blond, and proud.
She makes no apologies for her golden tresses. In her new black-
and-white music video, directed by Matthew Rolston, Mary J.
plays the role of a torch singer with the sweet sadness of a sepia
Jean Harlow. On "Soul Train," she wears her blond ponytail under
a bright red baseball cap and there's nothing wannabe about it.

Black women may not be natural blonds, but they do know how to
mix blondness with hip-hop attitude and blues-singer soul. Women
like Mary J. understand that beauty, like freedom, is about express-
ing dreams and possibilities. After all, it was Alice Walker who said,
"Oppressed hair puts a ceiling on the brain."

Veronica Chambers

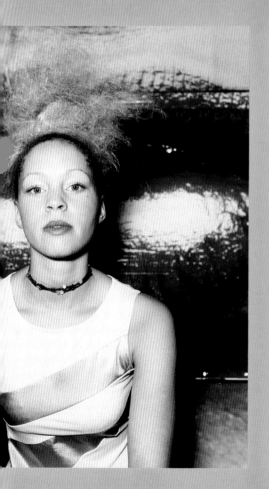

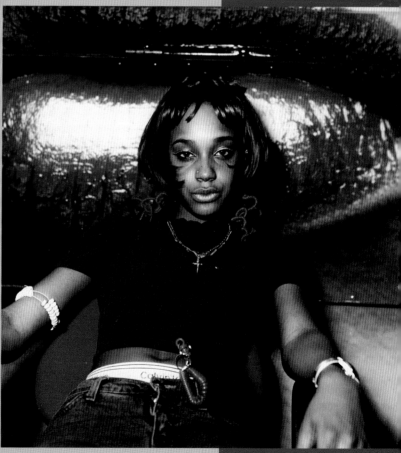

HAIR PEACE

All I want is flexibility and versatility. I would like to be able to do a lot of different things with my hair, and, as a black woman, I do have options: natural hair, permed/relaxed/texturized hair, short straight hair, short nappy hair, long nappy hair, braids, Senegalese twists, dreadlocks, pressed hair...the possibilities are endless, and when it comes to hairstyling black women are creative geniuses. I've seen our women wearing some of the most beautiful styles. But what I want mostly is healthy hair, whether it's long, short, natural, or straight. . . .

Hair is the black woman's obsession. Well, I want to stop obsessing over "what to do next" with my head and start channeling my energy into developing other parts of who I am. I love my hair, and I feel like I have really grown to accept and appreciate it.

Aliona L. Gibson

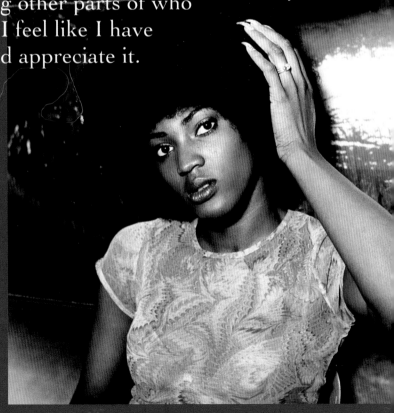

SOURCES

The author would like to thank the museums, collectors, libraries, models, and photographers for giving their kind permission for their images to be reproduced, and for their friendly support during the production of this book. All reasonable effort has been made to find and contact the copyright owners of the illustrations printed in this publication. Any omissions or errors are inadvertent.

Picture Credits

Front cover; Matthew Jordan Smith, *Portrait of Alva Rogers*. Courtesy LVA Photo Agency. © Matthew Jordan Smith. End Papers; Eileen Perrier, *Hair Products* from *The Black Hair and Beauty Show Project*, London. © Eileen Perrier.

4-5. Kevin Williams/WAK, *Doing Time* from *A Day at the Salon Series*. © Kevin Williams.

7-8. Winifred Hall Allen, 1900-1940. *Lilac Beauty Shop*. Courtesy Jeanne Moutoussamy-Ashe.

11. Winifred Hall Allen, 1900-1940. *Beauticians of the Ritz Beauty Shop*. Courtesy Jeanne Moutoussamy-Ashe.

12-13. Jacob Lawrence, *Rooftops (No.1, This is Harlem)* 1943. Gouache with pencil under drawing on paper. 15 3/8 x 1 11/16." © Courtesy of the estate of Jacob Lawrence & The Hirshhorn Museum and Sculpture Garden, Smithsonian Institution, 1966. Photograph by Lee Stalsworth.

14. Jesse Covington, *Album Quilt*, 1895-1900, 81 x 80." © Collection of Dr. and Mrs. Richard H. Hulan.

15. Paul Goodnight, *Links and Lineage*. Courtesy of the artist.

16. Kent Reno, Woman Combing Hair, Abidjan, Ivory Coast, 1980. Courtesy of the photographer. © Kent Reno

17. Carrie Mae Weems, *Woman Combing Hair*, from the Kitchen Table Series. Courtesy PPOW Gallery, New York. © Carrie Mae Weems.

19-20. Ruth Russell Williams, *The Kitchen Beautician*, 1993. Courtesy of Ruth Russell Williams. © Ruth Russell Williams.

21-22. Annie Lee, *You Next Sugar*. Courtesy of the artist.

25. Austin Hansen, *Students of Apex Beauty School Demonstrating Hairstyling and Nail Care*, 1970s. Used by permission of Joyce Hansen & The Schomburg Center for Research in Black Culture, New York

26-27. Eileen Perrier, *Perm Kit Gloves* from The Black Hair and Beauty Show Project, London.

28. Winifred Hall Allen, 1900-1940. *Mrs. Scott Owner of Ritz Shoppe* (seated in front). Courtesy Jeanne Moutoussamy-Ashe.

29. Unknown Photographer, *Mahalia Jackson Being Interviewed*. The Schomburg Center for Research in Black Culture, New York

30-31. Annie Lee, *Hot Comb*, 1994. Courtesy of Annie Lee.

33. Photograph by Edward Keating, *Classmates at School Prom*, 1994. © Edward Keating and New York Times

39. Gentl & Hyers, 1997. Courtesy Edge Photo Agency. © Gentl and Hyers.

40. Photograph by Matthew Jordan Smith. © Matthew Jordan Smith

40. Guglielmo Massaia, *Shawan Hairstyles for Mourning*, from *I miei trentacinque anni di missione nell' alta Etiopia*, 1885-95. Courtesy Robert Pankhurst.

41. Photograph by John Peden. ©John Peden

42-43. Annie Lee, *Spit, Shine and Fingerwave*

45. Nefertiti, *Getting Fixed to Look Pretty*, 1978. Linocut, 44 x 40" PR.87.014. Courtesy Schomburg Center for Research in Black Culture, The New York Public Library.

46. Photograph by Jeffrey Gamble, model: Tinuola Arowolo. Courtesy of the photographer. © Jeffrey Gamble.

47-48. Photograph by Daniel Green. Courtesy of the photographer. © Daniel Green.

49. Photograph by James Hicks, model: Fatou, New York Model Agency.

50. Photograph by Jeffrey Gamble, model: Liris Crosse, Wilhelmina Models, New York

51. Eve Arnold, *An African-American Woman Adjusting Wigs*, c. 1964. © Photograph by Eve Arnold/Magnum Photos.

52-53. Angela Fisher, *Guedra Dancer- Plaited hair embellished with pendant, carved shell disks, talismans and extra hair bun*. Courtesy of the Robert Estall Photo Agency, London © Angela Fisher.

58-62. Photograph by Austin Hansen, c.1940s. Used by permission of Joyce Hansen and the Schomburg Center for Research in Black Culture

63. *Painting of Lady Thepu (Tjepu)*. From Thebes, Tomb 181, New Kingdom, Dynasty XVIII, reign of Amunhotep III. Painted Plaster, Height: 11 7/8" (30.2cm) Brooklyn Museum of Art, Charles Wilbour Fund 65.197

65-66. Courtesy Bundles/Walker Family Collection

69. *Combs*. Back row, left to right: a. Akan, Ghana, wood; b. Somalia, wood; c. Zaire, reed, bamboo; d. Zaire, ivory; Zaire? Angola? Wood, metal; f. Tutsi, Rwanda, wood; g. Zaire, brass, iron. Front row, left to right: h. Nande, Zaire, wood, metal; i. Lega, Zaire, ivory; j. Pende, Zaire, wood; k. Luba, Zaire, wood, copper,wire; l. Asante, Ghana, wood; m. Baule, Ivory Coast, ivory; n. Yaka, Kwango River, Zaire, wood; o. Susu, Cowakry, Guinea, bamboo. © UCLA Fowler Museum of Cultural History. Photograph by Denis J. Nervig.

70-71. *Salon Kije barbershop sign*. Courtesy The Museum for African Art, New York

72-73. ©Photograph by Bob Adelman/Magnum Photos Inc

74. Photograph by Anthony Barboza. Courtesy of the photographer

78-79. Photograph by Eli Reed/Magnum Photos, Inc

80-81. Costa Manos/Magnum Photos, Inc

82. Hugh Grannum, *School Girl in Dakar, Senegal*, 1985. Courtesy of Hugh Grannum

83. Raymond Depardon, *New York Children Playing*. Harlem, New York, 1981. © Raymond Depardon/Magnum Photos, Inc.

84. *Standing Male Figure*, Ivory Coast, Baule. Wood, height 54.4.cm. Photograph by Mario Carrieri. Courtesy Estate of Carlo Monzino

85. Brent Jones, *Portrait of young girl* (First day of voluntary school integration, lone black girl on school bus), Milwaukee Wisconsin, 1976. Courtesy of Brent Jones. © Brent Jones.

87-91. Kevin Williams (WAK), *Hair Werks Posters*. c. 1970s. © Soft Sheen Inc

93. Photograph by Yusef Rashad. Courtesy of Yusef Rashad. © Yusef Rashad.

94-95. Eve Arnold, *Arlene Hawkins with Afro Puffs*. c. 1968. © Photograph by Eve Arnold/Magnum Photos, Inc

97. Melton Prior. *Sketch of Cape Coast (Ghana) Women's Hairstyles, Illustrated London News*, April 4, 1874.

99. Matthew Jordan Smith *Photograph of Alva Rogers*.

100. Photograph by Bruce Davidson. © Bruce Davidson/Magnum Photos, Inc

103-104. Chester Higgins, *Preparing for a Celebration*, Ghana, 1975. Courtesy of Chester Higgins. © Chester Higgins.

106. *Heddle Pulley*, Ivory Coast, Guro. Wood, height 16.5cm (right). Photograph by Mario Carrieri. Courtesy Estate of Carlo Monzino.

108-109. Amos Ferguson, *Mermaid*. International Folk Art Foundation Collection in the Museum of International Folk Art, a unit of the Museum of New Mexico, Santa Fe. Photograph by Blair Clark.

110-111. Annie Lee, *Extensions.*, 1998. Courtesy of Annie Lee. © Annie Lee.

112. Photograph by Joe Grant

115. Photograph by Terance Carney

118. Photograph by Preston Phillips

119. Photograph of Cornrow Hairstyle.°

122-123. Winifred Hall Allen (1900-1940), *A Hairstyle*. Courtesy © Jeanne Moutoussamy-Ashe

124. Seydou Keita, *Portrait of Senegalese Woman*. c. 1950s. Jean Pigozzi Collection. © CAAC/Keita.

125. Bruce Davidson, *Harlem Vote for Miss Beaux Arts*. c. 1963. © Bruce Davidson/Magnum Photos, Inc

126. Photograph by Norman Frederick (left)

126. *Heddle Pulley*, Ivory Coast, Guro. Wood height 16.5cm (right). Photograph by Mario Carrieri. Courtesy Estate of Carlo Monzino.

127. Angela Fisher, *Oromo Girl*. (Stylish woman at local market place in central Highlands, Welo Province, Ethiopia. Courtesy Robert Estall Photo Agency. © Angela Fisher.
127. Photograph by John Peden. © John Peden.
128-129. Photograph by Joseph Nevadomsky.
130. Bitok T. Pierre, *Catherine Hairdresser & Braider*. Photograph by Jean-Marie Lerat.
132-139. Bitok T. Pierre, *Untitled Hair Salon Sign*. Photograph by Jean-Marie Lerat.
140. Ruth Marten, *Fuquanda*. 1999. Courtesy of the artist. © Ruth Marten.
143-144. Eileen Perrier, *Untitled Portraits (The Black Hair and Beauty Show Project)*, London

° This photograph is reproduced here without explicit permission of the copyright holder(s). It is not my intention to violate any such copyrights. If you feel your rights are infringed in one way or another, please contact me immediately to find a way to settle any issues, in line with accepted illustrsated book publishing industry fees.

Text Credits

9. Hilton Als, "The Shop" (excerpt) from *The New York Times Magazine*. April 6, 1997. Courtesy of the author.
14. Julie Dash, (excerpt) from *Daughter's of the Dust: The Making of an African American Woman's Film* by Julie Dash. The New Press, NY, 1992. Courtesy of the author
16. Bell Hooks, (excerpt) from *Daughter's of the Dust: The Making of an African American Woman's Film* by Julie Dash. The New Press, NY, 1992. Courtesy of Bell Hooks
17. Henry Louis Gates, Jr., "It All Comes Down to the Kitchen" (excerpt) from *Colored People* by Henry Louis Gates, Jr., Copyright ©1994 by Henry Louis Gates, Jr. Reprinted by permission of Alfred A. Knopf, a division of Random House, Inc.
18. Bell Hooks, (excerpt) from *Daughter's of the Dust: The Making of an African American Woman's Film* by Julie Dash. The New Press, NY, 1992. Courtesy of Bell Hooks
21. Pauletta Lewis, (excerpt) from *Poetic Justice: Fimmaking South Central Style* by John Singleton and Veronica Chambers; foreword by Spike Lee. Delta Press, New York 1993.
23. Sheneska Jackson, (excerpt) from *Blessings*, by Sheneska Jackson. Scribner, New York 1999. Sheneska Jackson. Copyright © 1998 Sheneska Jackson. Courtesy of the author.
24. Natasha Trethewey "Naola Beauty Academy" from *Domestic Work* by Natasha Trethewey. Greystone Press New York, 2000. Courtesy of the author.
31. Natasha Trethewey "Hot Comb" from *Domestic Work* by Natasha Trethewey. Greystone Press New York, 2000. Courtesy of the author.
32. Gwendolyn Brooks "Gimme an upsweep Minnie" from *Blacks* by Gwendolyn Brooks. Third World Press, Chicago 1991. Copyright © Courtesy of the estate of Gwendolyn Brooks.
39. Willie Coleman "Among the Things That Use to Be" from *Home Girls: A Black Feminist Anthology*, ed. Barbara Smith, Kitchen Table: Women of Color Press, 1983. Courtesy of Willie Colelman

42-43. Sharan Strange "Barbershop Ritual" from *In The Tradition: An Anthology of Young Black Writers* eds. By kevin Powell and Ras Baraka. Harlem River Press, New York 1992. Copyright © 1990 by Sharan Strange.
44. Karen Williams "Beauty Shop" Courtesy of Karen Williams, 2001.
46-50. Daryle Bennett interview, April 25, 2001. Copyright © Ima Ebong, 2001.
52. Angela Fisher "Guedra Dancer" caption from *Africa Adorned* by Angela Fisher. Harvill Press, London, 1987. Copyright © Angela Fisher.
54-57. George C. Wolfe "Battle of the Wigs,' from *The Colored Museum* by George C. Wolfe. Copyright © 1985. 1987, 1988 by George C. Wolfe. Used by permission of Grove/Atlantic, Inc.
63. Michael Sones "Hair in Ancient Egypt" (excerpt) from Beautyworlds.com. Courtesy of Editor, Beautyworlds.com. www.Beautyworlds.com.
64. Langston Hughes "Wigs, Women and Falsies," from *Langston Hughes: The Return of Simple*, ed., by Akiba Sullivan Harper, Introduction by Arnold Rampersad. Hill and Wang, New York, 1995. © Estate of Langston Hughes.
72. Maria Galati "Nappy Head" from *Quiet Storm: Voices of Young Black Poets*, Selected by Lydia Omolola Okutoro. Copyright © 1999 by Lydia Omolola Okutoto. Used by permission of Hyperion Books, New York 1999.
73. Stacy Lyn Evans "Good Hair" from *Real Soul Food & other poetic recipes*, by Stacey Lyn Evans. Copyright © 1995 by Stacy Lyn Evans. Used by permission of Black Words, Alexandria, VA 2000.
74. Kelly M. Page "Halo" from *Quiet Storm: Voices of Young Black Poets*, Selected by Lydia Omolola Okutoro. Copyright © 1999 by Lydia Omolola Okutoto. Used by permission of Hyperion Books, New York 1999.
75. Harriet Jacobs "On Extending the Olive Branch to my own Self" from *Spirit & Flame: An Anthology of Contemporary African American Poetry*, ed. Keith Gilyard. Copyright © by Hariett Jacobs. Used by permission of Syracuse University Press, Syracuse, New York 1997.
77. Gwendolyn Brooks "To Those of My Sisters Wearing Natural Hair," from *Blacks* by Gwendolyn Brooks. Third World Press, Chicago 1991. Copyright © The Estate of Gwendolyn Brooks.
78. Maxine Tynes "Borrowed Beauty" from *Daughters of the Sun Women of the Moon: Poetry by Black Canadian Women*. Ed., by Ann Wallace. Africa World Press, Inc., New Jersey 1991. Courtesy of Maxine Tynes.
80. Linda G. Hardnett "If Hair Makes Me Black, I Must Be Purple" from *A Galaxy of Black Writing*. Ed., R. Baird Shuman. Moore Publishing Company, Durham, North Carolina 1971. Used by Permission of R. Baird Shuman.
81. Debraha Watson "Good Hair," Copyright © Debraha Watson, 1994.
83. Monifa Atungaye Love "Initiation I" excerpt from *In Search of Color Everywhere: A Collection of African-American Poetry*, ed., by

E. Ethelbert Miller. Stewart, Tabori & Chang, New York 1994. Courtesy of Monifa Atungaye Love
86. Lois Griffith "By the Hair" from *Aloud: Voices from the Nuyorican Poets' Café*, ed., by Miguel Algarin and Bob Colman. Owlet Press, New York 1994.
92. Crystal Williams "Dreadlock," from *Kin* by Crystal Williams. Michigan State University Press, East Lansing, Michigan 2000. Courtesy of Crystal Williams.
93. Tracie Morris "Rasta Not" from *Intermission* by Tracie Morris. Soft Skull Press, New York 1998. Courtesy of Tracie Morris.
95. Tracie Morris "A Hair Poem of Black Girls" from *Intermission* by Tracie Morris. Soft Skull Press, New York 1998. Courtesy of Tracie Morris
95. Gwendolyn Brooks "Southeast Corner" from *Blacks* by Gwendolyn Brooks. Third World Press, Chicago 1991. Copyright © The Estate of Gwendolyn Brooks. Used by permission of The Gwendolyn Brooks Estate.
96. Charlotte Watson Sherman "Roots" from *In Search of Color Everywhere: A Collection of African-American Poetry*, ed., by E. Ethelbert Miller. Stewart, Tabori & Chang, New York 1994. Courtesy of Charlotte Watson Sherman.
96. Melton Prior "Female Fashions at Cape Coast Castle" from *London Illustrated News*, April 4, 1874.
98. Jennifer McLune "My First Love" from *Quiet Storm: Voices of Young Black Poets*, Selected by Lydia Omolola Okutoro. Copyright © 1999 by Lydia Omolola Okutoro. Used by permission of Hyperion Books, New York 1999.
99. Maya Angelou "My Hair, a Hive of Honey Bees" from *Now Sheba Sings* by Maya Angelou, Illustrated by Tom Feelings. Dutton/Dial Books, New York. 1987. Courtesy Maya Angelou.
101. Karen Williams "There's History in my Hair" from *Spirit & Flame: An Anthology of Contemporary African American Poetry*, ed. Keith Gilyard. Copyright © by Hariett Jacobs. Used by permission of Syracuse University Press, Syracuse, New York 1997.
104. Karen Williams. "Hair: The Filament of Life." Copyright © Karen Williams, 1998. Courtesy of Karen Williams. Annu Prestonia interview, April 27, 2001. Copyright © Ima Ebong, 2001. "Oromo Girl" caption, from *Africa Adorned* by Angela Fisher. Harvill Press, London,1987. Copyright © Angela Fisher.
131. Jean-Marie Lerat "Advertising Art Adorns African Cities." Copyright © Jean-Marie Lerat.
137-138. Nina Gwatkin, (excerpt) from *Yoruba Hairstyles: A Selection of Hairstyles from Southern Nigeria* by Nina W. Gwatkin, Photographs by Ann Goodall. The Craft Centre, National Museum Lagos, Nigeria, 1971. "caption
142. Veronica Chambers "Blonde Like Me," *New York Times Magazine*. © Veronica Chambers.
144. Aliona L. Gibson "Hair Peace" (excerpt) from *Nappy: Growing Up Black and Female in America*, by Aliona L. Gibson, Harlem River Press, New York 1995. Courtesy Aliona Gibson. © Aliona Gibson.